MAKING YOUR OWN COSMETICS

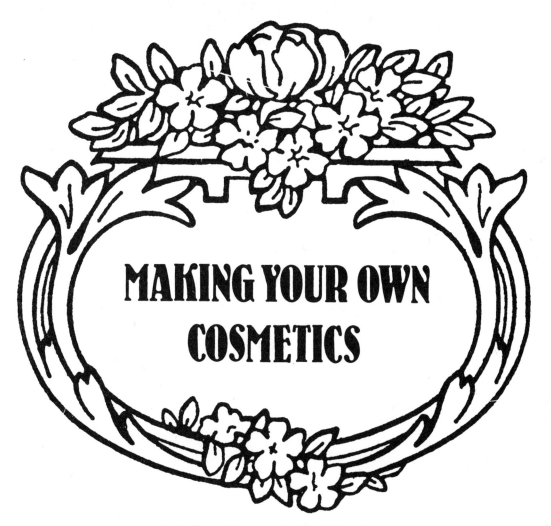

MAKING YOUR OWN COSMETICS

including make-up; perfumes; hair; skin-care
and personal hygiene preparations
for men and women; aromatherapy

James Sholto Douglas

PELHAM BOOKS
LONDON

To Mary

First published in Great Britain by
PELHAM BOOKS LTD
52 Bedford Square
London WC1B 3EF
1979

ISBN 0 7207 1042 1

Filmset in Great Britain by
Northumberland Press Ltd, Gateshead, Tyne and Wear.
Printed by Hollen Street Press,
141 Farnham Road, Slough, Bucks.

Contents

Acknowledgements

The author wishes to express his gratitude to the following
individuals and organizations for their kind help and per-
mission to reproduce material: the Editor of *Soap, Perfumery and Cosmetics*; the Editor of *The Flavour Industry*;
Dragoco (Great Britain) Ltd; the Editor of *The Gardener's
Chronicle*; the Editor of *Essential Oil and Perfumery
Record*.

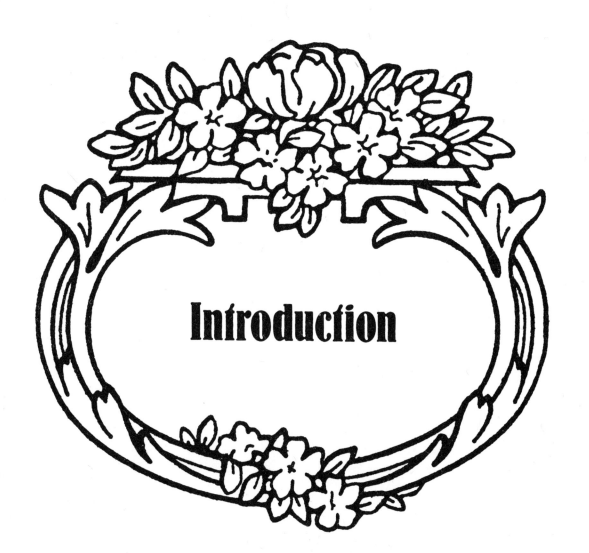

Introduction

There are several important reasons why we should all try to make at home as many of our own cosmetics, toiletries and perfumes as possible. First, it is now very expensive to buy most of these preparations – indeed the prices of many of the better-quality products are so high that they may well be more than the cost of their equivalent weight in gold. Second, increasing quantities of synthetic materials and different chemicals are being used in the manufacture of proprietary cosmetics and toilet articles. Just as mass-produced food-stuffs are adulterated today, so also may be the beauty and health aids and preparations that we use regularly. Third, it is not very difficult to make excellent cosmetics and toiletries in your own home; only a small amount of time and little effort are required and you will have the satisfaction of knowing that what you are using is generally pure and good for the skin, the hair and the body. There is no effective substitute for natural products. Home-made cosmetics are to a great extent compounded from materials obtained from natural or related sources, such as essential and fixed oils, preparations of herbs and other plants, fruit extracts, waxes, honey, fats, lanolin, different minerals and earths and gums, or their derivatives. Some of these substances have been known and used for thousands of years as aids to hygiene and beauty.

My work with plants over many years has shown me that a very wide range of useful and health-giving commodities can be obtained with little trouble or difficulty from different species which, if exploited properly and made available directly to the public, would provide better-quality, cheaper goods. In the case of cosmetics and toilet preparations, some of the main ingredients such as oils and fats are derived from plants and can be bought in the pure form at a fraction of the cost of purchasing a ready-made formula or product.

8

Perfumes and scents are chiefly composed of essential or ethereal oils of various types, yielded by trees and shrubs or other crops, blended together and expensively labelled.

This book sets out to show readers what cosmetics are, how they can be prepared at home, and the different ingredients that should be used to make satisfactory beauty aids and toiletries at less cost. I hope it will be helpful and valuable to both women and men. The care and protection of our skins, hair and bodies is a vital and necessary task, complementary to the attention that we give to our diet and hygiene.

Cosmetics include not only preparations designed to clean or beautify the face and body, but also items used for hygiene purposes such as dentifrices, toilet waters and powders, shampoos, shaving soaps, antiperspirants and deodorants, and scents and perfumes. In fact it may be said that all products for application to the body that help to make the user look or feel more attractive and acceptable to others come under the category of cosmetics.

Efficacious and useful though cosmetics and toiletries are, it must be remembered that there is no real substitute for good soap and water for cleansing purposes. Only if there are medical reasons for not using soap should this important fact be neglected. Before reading the detailed instructions for making your own cosmetics, careful attention should be paid to these points:

(a) Where fruit and vegetables are specified in formulae or for different purposes, always use fresh ones. Never substitute canned or frozen fruits or vegetables for any treatments because they will not necessarily possess the same qualities and may contain added sugar, preservatives or chemicals of some kind or other.

(b) Certain people may be allergic to various products. If

9

you are allergic to a particular ingredient in any cosmetic, do not use it. It may cause skin irritation or illness.

(c) As you read this book, try to become familiar with the special properties of different commodities. Some of the listed products are mild bleaches, others have soothing and moisturizing attributes, while in special instances health-giving effects may be expected.

So now to work. Making your own cosmetics at home will not only save you money and give you greater satisfaction and pleasure, but it also constitutes a profitable and interesting occupation and a rewarding pastime.

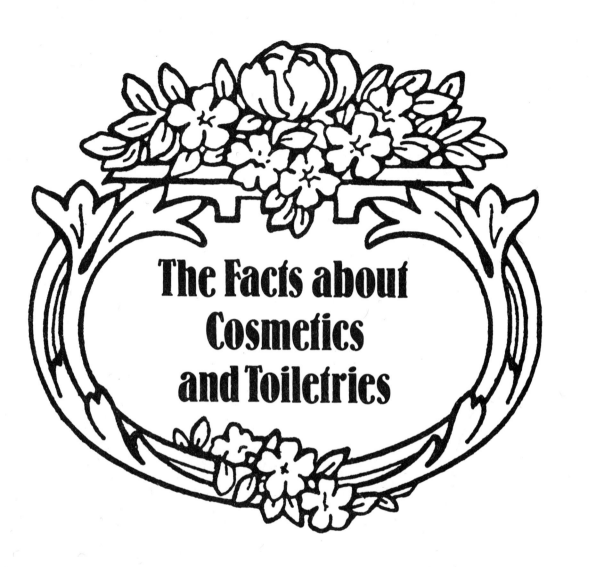

The Facts about Cosmetics and Toiletries

The word 'cosmetics' is derived from the Greek verb *kosmeein*, to adorn or embellish. From the Latin *tela,* meaning a web, we have received the term 'toiletries', relating to items or articles used in dressing or to perfect a person's appearance and cleanliness. The main object of all cosmetics and toilet preparations is to render the user more beautiful and pleasing to others; in that sense they may be said to act as webs to catch the attention and interest of friends, colleagues and bystanders. As the poet Alexander Pope (1688–1744) wrote in *The Rape of the Lock:*

> Fair tresses man's imperial race insnare,
> And beauty draws us with a single hair...

so does everyone think when confronted with a well turned-out person. It is therefore natural to try to improve and maintain one's looks with the help of cosmetics properly and skilfully applied.

History of beauty aids

The use of cosmetics dates back for thousands of years to very ancient times. Evidence of the employment of eye make-up and various aromatic ointments has been found in Egyptian tombs of 3500 BC. In those days, perfumes and scents obtained from plants were greatly esteemed and were often reserved for religious ceremonies. In the New Testament we read how Mary Magdalene poured on to the head of Jesus the contents of a precious box of ointment of spikenard, an aromatic oil or balsam yielded by the Indian valerian plant. Kohl, a fine powder of antimony, was employed in the East for staining the eyelids, while the Assyrians used a blue

12

preparation for the same purpose. It was considered that this colour minimized the harmful effect of strong sunlight. Amongst the ladies of the Roman Empire it was quite common to bleach the hair or wear wigs. Lipstick, eyeshadow and rouge were well known and perfumes were popular. In classical Greece, too, scents were in use and cheeks were reddened with alkanet, obtained from the roots of a Mediterranean plant. More unhappily white lead, a poisonous substance, was used for whitening the skin. In the Arab countries henna has always been esteemed. It is used to dye the hair and nails and is produced by a small shrub of the loosestrife family which bears fragrant white flowers. The pigment comes from the leaves.

In addition to these facial cosmetics, abrasive powders or dentifrices were used to clean the teeth, and there were scented unguents and different oils which were used while bathing and for rubbing into the body, especially the legs and arms. Popular oils included those obtained from almonds and olives. Essential oils were produced from various aromatic plants and formed the constituents of perfumes with spicy or floral fragrances. Natural gums or resins were employed as perfumery fixatives.

When the western Roman Empire fell in the fifth century AD, much of Europe lapsed into barbarism although the eastern part of the Empire, together with India, Persia and China, continued to maintain cultured and civilized life. In these areas, the development of the art of cosmetics continued, but it was not until the thirteenth century, after the end of the Dark Ages and the coming of the Crusades, that cosmetics were reintroduced into the West. Perfumes for adornment, hair dyes, facial cosmetics, and toiletries for the bath and general health again became known to the wealthier sections of the population and were used whenever possible.

The end of the nineteenth century and the first half of the twentieth saw considerable advances in the production of commercial cosmetics. Among new inventions were the collapsible tube, the cold permanent wave and soapless shampoos, aerosol containers and special hair colorants.

It must not be forgotten that cosmetics were by no means confined to women. Facial decoration for men has always been associated with war and magic. The warpaint of North American Indians was justly famous and similar examples may be seen in the remoter districts of Papua. In Africa, the male face is frequently painted for participation in ritual and tribal dances, as well as for witchcraft. Hair-styling is also well developed amongst Africans and the use of certain oils for hair dressings is fully understood.

The Asian countries were for long the chief producers of scent oils, mainly because many of the plants yielding these essences grow in Asia. The use of perfumes was widespread in India during the time of the Mogul Empire. In China, too, many valuable plant species were known and used for the extraction of aromatic materials. Other important growing localities were the East Indies, formerly called the Spice Islands, and the Philippines.

The range of cosmetics

Any full list of cosmetic preparations is necessarily long, but for convenience it is possible to group the different kinds of beauty aids into quite well defined classes according to the purposes for which they are used.

For skin-care   In this section we have first of all *cleansing creams* and *cleansing lotions,* which are important for cleaning the skin especially if it is sensitive to soap or if make-up has to be removed. Such preparations are generally composed of oils, which act as solvents, mixed with water to form an emulsion. The consistency can vary from that of thick cold cream to a relatively thin cleansing milk. Solutions of herbs in water are also used for cleaning and stimulating the skin.

Softening creams or *emollients,* the so-called night creams and nourishing or moisturizing creams, are actually heavier types of cold cream. These may be massaged into the skin and some left on the face as a thick film overnight to minimize the loss of moisture.

Hand creams and *hand lotions* are intended to prevent dryness and roughness of the skin on the hands and they act largely by replacing lost moisture and providing an oily, protective film. They are often made up as oil-in-water emulsions.

Tonics and *fresheners* are dilute alcoholic lotions containing astringents and possibly germicides.

For make-up *Foundations* include *vanishing cream,* an oil-in-water emulsion containing stearic acid – a solid fatty acid – a small part of which is saponified (made into soap); and *liquid foundations* with less oil but some pigment or colouring.

Face powder is made commercially from talc, chalk or kaolin, materials such as magnesium stearate, zinc oxide and titanium dioxide, and various pigments to give different colours.

Rouge is a mixture of colour and talc or fats and waxes employed to redden the face. Blushers are used increasingly today.

Eye make-up includes *mascara* for the eyelashes, *eye shadow* for the eyelids, and *eyebrow pencils* and *eyeliner* to pick out the edges of the lids.

Lipstick has a fatty base which, although firm in itself, spreads easily. The colour is provided by pigments or stains. *Lip salves* have little or no colour and protect the lips by a fairly thick fatty coating against wind, sun and aridity. They may also provide a glossy finish.

Sunscreens – specific sunscreen ingredients may be incorporated in some suitable oil or cream to give a protective film over the skin when sunbathing. They enable you to tan but prevent burning.

For the hair Modern *shampoos* have as their basis a negatively charged detergent of good solubility, unaffected by hard water and with high grease-removing properties. Soap alone may cause considerable scum. Shampoos may contain special ingredients to check dandruff or for dry or greasy hair. Various saponaceous plants provide leaves, twigs or stems that yield good lather for shampooing when rubbed in water; these are natural sources of hair cleansers.

Hairdressings include proprietary sets and sprays. Simple hair sprays may be composed of a natural resin such as shellac, with some perfume, dissolved in alcohol, a volatile solvent. Both sexes use these sprays, which are applied by aerosol. Hair used to be set with gum solutions, normally of tragacanth, which is effective and quite cheap. These *gominas* are particularly popular in Latin America. There are many oily dressings which give a gloss to hair and fix it in place to some extent. *Brilliantines* are composed of nearly one hundred per cent oily matter, but *emulsions* are mixtures of water and oil. Curly and wavy hair is best controlled by emulsions because the water makes the hair easier to style in the first place. Brilliantines or *pomades,* on the other hand, suit straight hair or short, frizzy hair which does not need restyling. In Asia and Africa locally-produced natural oils,

16

especially coconut oil, are popular and easily available for hairdressing. The bases of heavy, thick brilliantines and pomades are petroleum oils and jellies, to which are added some scent and colouring.

Alcoholic lotions for the hair give a fresh feeling and stimulus to the scalp and are popular in Europe and South America. Hair *conditioners* and *strengtheners* are supposed to improve out-of-condition hair, caused chiefly by the effects of environmental pollution, excessive combing, bleaching and setting and colouring, with consequent surface damage to the scales.

Hair colorants and bleaches cover up grey, mousy or dull hair. There are many proprietary products in the shops, as well as some natural sources.

For fragrance *Perfumes* and *scents* may be found in virtually all cosmetic preparations. Fragrances are normally divided into three types of *notes,* called *top, middle* and *base.* Top notes provide the more volatile, immediate kind of odours. Middle notes should give a full, solid character to a scent. Base notes are responsible for less volatile, more persistent smells.

In commercial preparations the ingredients producing the fragrances may be of plant, animal or chemical origin. A simple essence can be made from twenty or more constituents, and a good proprietary perfume may contain over one hundred ingredients – often, however, quite unnecessarily.

In practice the most straightforward fragrances are *toilet waters,* which are mixtures of aqueous alcohol with small proportions of scent-producing ingredients, often fugitive or short-lived, but which give a fresh feeling on impact with the skin. More concentrated perfumes are actually solutions of the essence in question with alcohol, and much attention is paid by manufacturers to the creation of high-class and expensive scents.

Fragrance vehicles are made of alcohol gelled with soap and suitably perfumed, for instance cologne sticks. They are solid or semi-solid.

For hygiene *Dentifrices* contain some kind of abrasive for scouring the teeth, together with a vehicle to carry this material, and suitable flavouring. Here is a typical toothpaste formula:

	% in mixture
Calcium phosphate, chalk, alumina	40
Glycerine	20
Sodium lauryl sulphate (detergent)	1·5
Thickener (sodium carboxymethyl cellulose)	1
Flavour	1
Water	36·5
Total	100

It is quite common today for fluorides such as salt of hydrofluoric acid or fluorophosphates to be added to dentifrices. They are said to fight dental decay, but their efficacy depends very much upon the skill of the formulator in preserving the activity of the added fluorine compounds.

Mouthwashes normally have a mild germicidal action and leave a pleasant taste in the mouth.

Antiperspirants and deodorants – the safest and most effective commercial antiperspirants are made from aluminium derivatives. Deodorants are really mild germicides with some perfume added. Popular sprays and roll-on applicators may combine an antiperspirant to reduce sweating, a deodorant to lessen odour, and a scent to give a pleasant smell.

Bath preparations include germicidal soaps, bath crystals and oils, and bubble and foam baths. All these items may scent the skin and produce a feeling of well-being after use. *Bath salts* or *bath cubes* for dissolving in bath water also have a softening effect and reduce soap scum.

Talcum and dusting powders and *after-bath preparations* are generally aids to body freshness and are very popular. *Alcoholic lotions* and *cologne waters* are also much used for hygiene purposes. Sometimes talcum powders contain small amounts of germicide to reduce the odour of perspiration, thus having a deodorizing effect.

Depilatories are used to remove body hair. The active ingredient in these creams or pastes is often calcium thioglycollate, which weakens the hairs so that they can be removed at skin level with little effort. Waxes can be used, too, which set around the hairs and allow them to be pulled out of the follicles when the wax is removed.

For miscellaneous purposes Under this section come *shaving preparations,* made up as soaps, creams and foams, brushless creams, pre-shave lotions and powders and aftershave lotions. To make shaving easy and pleasant the beard must be moistened to soften it. This takes three to four minutes, which means that a *shaving cream, soap* or *foam* should have a consistency or lather to hold water in contact with the hair for that time. The foam produced by soaps, sticks and creams should be tight and slow to collapse. *Brushless creams* give a similar result without lathering. They are rather like foundation vanishing creams, being oil-in-water emulsions.

Pre-shave lotions and *powders* are used to prepare the face for dry shaving with an electric razor.

Aftershave preparations are alcoholic, rather less scented than ordinary colognes and often include astringents which are supposed to tone up the skin and leave a fresh feeling. Sometimes, however, they produce a burning or sore sensation on certain types of skin.

Manicure preparations are for the nails on hands and feet, and include *nail varnish* or lacquer and *removers*. Nail cosmetics are basically solutions of nitrocellulose lacquer mixed with plasticizers and colouring matter. Removers are solvents such as acetone and ethyl acetate.

Baby preparations are milder and less strongly-scented cosmetics, which should be completely free from any irritant substances.

Skin-lightening preparations are normally creams which contain hydroquinone or related chemicals that are claimed to have an effect upon the melanin or dark brown pigment in the skin.

Hair straighteners are products that straighten crinkly or fuzzy hair for a time. They should be used with great care.

Soaps – there are hundreds of different kinds of manufactured soaps. It is also quite practicable to make good soap at home.

Aromatherapy

The term aromatherapy refers mainly to the use of essential or ethereal oils – the same as those employed for making scents and perfumes – for the general care of the body. The oils are normally massaged gently into the skin to alleviate tiredness and fatigue. Fixed oils are used for similar treatments. The value of applying different oils to the body has been known and appreciated for thousands of years in many parts of the world.

Producing natural oils

Oil-yielding plants grow in abundance in most areas; in fact you can see some in most gardens. They can be easily and cheaply cultivated. To produce your own supply of oils is therefore not difficult because a simple still can be bought or made at home which will give excellent results.

Equipment

Making cosmetics at home has never required any great outlay or much time and labour. Lists of materials and where to obtain them will be found at the end of the book. Most of the jobs to be done are simply those of mixing and blending the ingredients. Remember that, to get good and uncontaminated products, you must take care to keep everything clean; the equipment should be thoroughly washed whenever you prepare a new batch. If you do not want to put chemical preservatives in those home-made preparations that have only a short life, store them in a refrigerator. However, many home-made items will keep indefinitely provided they are put in stoppered bottles or closed containers. Here again, make sure that the bottles or containers are clean beforehand, preferably by washing them in boiled water or even sterilizing them in a pan with boiling water for a few minutes, provided there is no danger of the material from which they are made cracking.

The chief items of equipment you will need for preparing cosmetics at home are more or less those that will be found in most kitchens:

Kitchen scales
Wooden spoons
Mixing bowls and/or blender/mixer
Thick saucepans and a double boiler
Ordinary teaspoons, tablespoons and knives
Bowls or basins and cups
Measures for fluid ounces and pints
Strainer and sieve
Thermometer – high-temperature, immersion type
Cotton gauze and muslin bags
Filter papers (optional)
Bottles, jars and other containers for storage.

Note All measures in the following recipes are in ounces or fluid ounces unless otherwise stated.

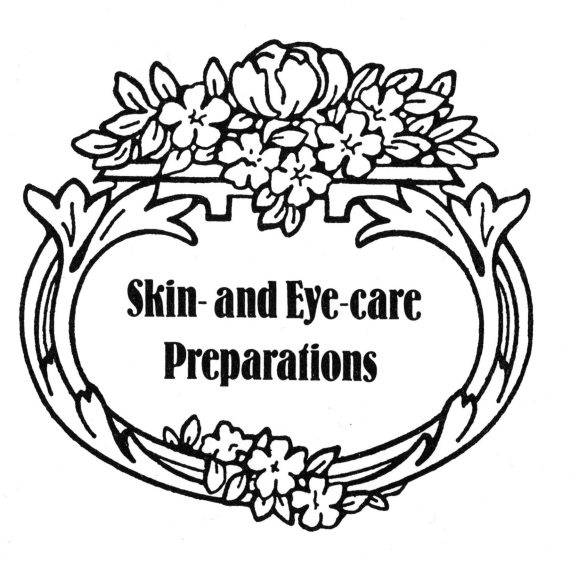

Skin- and Eye-care Preparations

Cleansing and cold creams

Although thorough washing with soap and water will clean the skin and remove surface grime, make-up and oil, there are certain advantages to be gained from using cleansing creams and lotions. They may get rid of dirt and stale make-up more readily, clear away solidified sebum or plaque and have a softening and protective effect on dry skin. In addition, any possible irritation caused by soap will be avoided.

The first known cold cream was prepared by the Greek doctor Galen who lived in Rome during the second century AD, though it is thought that he might have obtained the formula from Hippocrates (460–370 BC), the father of modern medicine. Before trying any of the following recipes you should read the general advice starting on page 14.

Galen's cold cream

	parts
Purified beeswax	1
Olive oil (in which rose petals have been macerated)*	3–4

Method Place the beeswax in a pan, heat it until it is liquid, then add the olive oil and mix well. Allow the mixture to cool and then blend in as much water as possible, so that a good cream results.

*To macerate means to soak or steep a substance in a liquid, if necessary for several days. Rose-scented oil or rose-perfumed water can be prepared by leaving the fragrant petals in the liquid until it has absorbed the rose scent.

This early cold cream was popular because it gave a pleasant, cool feeling and acted more rapidly and effectively than ordinary pomades made from fats or oils alone. In fact, it is the evaporation of water from skin cleansing creams that produces this cooling sensation.

In the course of time, to ensure better keeping qualities, more stability and whiteness and a softer cream, changes in the formula were made.

French cold cream

	parts		parts
White beeswax	12	Rosewater	$37\frac{1}{2}$
Almond oil	50		

Method Warm the beeswax and when it is liquid mix in the almond oil. Blend the rosewater slowly with this mixture to form a smooth cream.

In the above two recipes the parts listed may be measured out in any suitable way, such as ounces, grammes, spoonfuls or other weights and measures to suit the maker. For smaller amounts reduce the quantities, keeping the relative proportions equal.

Improved cold creams

(a) British

	parts		parts
White beeswax	9	Rosewater	10
Almond oil	$30\frac{1}{2}$	Rose oil	$\frac{1}{8}$
Borax	$\frac{1}{2}$		

Method Warm the beeswax and when it is liquid mix in the almond oil. Now dissolve the borax in the rosewater, heating it gently if necessary, and add it, stirring constantly, to the mixture of beeswax and almond oil. Finally add the rose oil and continue to stir until cool and the cream is well formed and blended.

(b) American

White beeswax	6	Rosewater	$2\frac{1}{2}$
Spermaceti	$6\frac{1}{4}$	Water	7
Almond oil	28	Rose oil	$\frac{1}{8}$
Borax	$\frac{1}{4}$		

Method Dissolve the borax in the water. Warm the beeswax and spermaceti, add the almond oil and then blend in the rosewater and the water in which the borax has been dissolved. Add the rose oil to this mixture and stir until cool.

All the cold creams mentioned so far should be kept in a refrigerator, because they may go rancid if left at room temperature for some time. The creams will keep better if you substitute mineral oil.

Cold cleansing cream

Beeswax	$8\frac{1}{4}$	Water	$16\frac{1}{4}$
Mineral oil	25	Any perfume oil	$\frac{1}{8}$
Borax	$\frac{1}{2}$		

Method Melt the beeswax in a pan and mix in mineral oil. Dissolve the borax in the water and add to the mixture of beeswax and mineral oil, stirring well as it cools. Then add the perfume oil. Continue blending until well creamed, and then cool.

26

Other cold cleansing creams

(a) Formulated for hot climates

Beeswax	$5\frac{3}{4}$	Mineral oil	$8\frac{1}{2}$
Spermaceti	$1\frac{1}{4}$	Borax	$\frac{1}{2}$
Carnauba wax	$2\frac{1}{2}$	Water	$15\frac{3}{4}$
Petroleum jelly (Vaseline or petrolatum)	16	Perfume oil	$\frac{1}{8}$

Method   Warm the beeswax, spermaceti and carnauba wax with the petroleum jelly, then add the mineral oil, blending well, followed by the water with the borax dissolved in it, and the perfume oil. Mix into a good cream and cool.

(b)

Beeswax	8	Borax	$\frac{1}{4}$
Mineral oil	$22\frac{1}{2}$	Water	$16\frac{1}{4}$
Paraffin wax	5	Perfume oil	$\frac{1}{8}$
Microcrystalline wax	$3\frac{1}{2}$		

Method   Melt the beeswax, paraffin wax and microcrystalline wax, then add the mineral oil, mix well and blend in the water in which the borax has already been dissolved. Work into a smooth cream, add the perfume oil, and cool.

(c)

Vegetable oil	$27\frac{1}{2}$	Water	$14\frac{3}{4}$
Beeswax	$7\frac{1}{4}$	Perfume oil	$\frac{1}{8}$
Borax	$\frac{1}{2}$		

Method   Warm the beeswax and mix with the vegetable oil,

then add the water in which the borax has already been dissolved. Add the perfume oil, blend into the cream and cool.

(d)

Vegetable oil	30	Borax	$\frac{1}{4}$
Spermaceti	1	Water	$11\frac{1}{4}$
Beeswax	$7\frac{1}{2}$	Perfume oil	$\frac{1}{8}$

Method Melt the beeswax and spermaceti, mix with the vegetable oil and then blend in the water in which the borax has been dissolved. Add the perfume oil, stirring until cool.

(e)

Vegetable oil	28	Zinc oxide	1
Beeswax	9	Water	$10\frac{1}{2}$
Lanolin	1	Perfume oil	$\frac{1}{8}$
Borax	$\frac{1}{2}$		

Method Prepare as for *(d)* above, melting the solid ingredients and blending in the oil, the water with the borax dissolved in it and perfume oil. Work into a cream and cool.

The term vegetable oil covers a variety of oils, any or a combination of which can be used. Suggested choices are peanut or groundnut oil, maize oil, wheatgerm oil, cottonseed oil, sunflower-seed oil, soya or soya bean oil, sesame or teel oil and similar products.

(f)

Beeswax	5	Borax	$\frac{1}{2}$
Mineral oil	27	Water	$12\frac{1}{2}$
Ozokerite	5	Perfume oil	$\frac{1}{8}$

Method Melt the solid ingredients and blend in the oil, the water with the borax dissolved in it and the perfume oil. Work into a cream and cool.

(*g*)

Beeswax	8	Borax	$\frac{1}{4}$
Mineral oil	$24\frac{1}{2}$	Water	$17\frac{1}{4}$
Paraffin wax	$3\frac{1}{2}$	Perfume oil	$\frac{1}{8}$
Cetyl alcohol	$\frac{1}{2}$		

Method Dissolve the borax in the water. Melt the solid ingredients, then add in the oil and other items. Stir continuously, add the perfume oil and work into a good cream.

General comments for preparation Mixing fats and oils and water when making cleansing cold creams involves the process of emulsification – that is to say, the combining of one or more liquids in others to form what are called 'suspensions'. It is important to add the water quite slowly to the fats and oils. Thorough stirring is also essential. Softened or distilled water is preferable to tap water, especially if you live in a hard-water area. Impure, undrinkable water should not be used. If you mix poorly, patches of water will remain in the cream, which will then consist of multiple emulsions instead of one well-blended, smooth, consistent emulsion. The best temperature for warming and melting the waxes and blending the oils is 158°–167°F (70°–75°C). When this temperature has been reached and the water blended in to form the emulsion, cool the mixture slowly and continue to stir it slowly until it reaches a temperature of 104°–113°F

(40°–45°C). The perfume oil can now be added. Go on stirring until just before the mixture starts to set, so that while still warm and semi-liquid it can be poured into jars and left to get cold.

Warning Remember that all the oily substances used in these recipes, such as beeswax, boil at very low temperatures and must be watched carefully. It is advisable to keep young children well away from the work area to eliminate the risk of accidents.

Preserving To preserve all cold creams and cleansing creams, the following substances can be added when the perfume oil is included: methyl parahydroxybenzoate at the rate of $\frac{1}{3}$ ounce to each 50 ounces of cream; or propyl parahydroxybenzoate at the rate of $\frac{1}{12}$ ounce to each 50 ounces of cream. Because the latter amount is such a small quantity it is easier to take a tiny portion of the preservative on the tip of a matchstick, which will be a fair measure.

Cleansing lotions and milks

Complexion cleansing lotions and milks, as well as liquid creams, have been used for many years under names such as *laits de beauté*, *laits de toilette*, or *laits virginals*. At first these lotions were made up from mixtures of soap, glycerine, witchhazel extract or rosewater to which were added alcoholic tinctures of gums such as benzoin or resins such as styrax and myrrh. Later, oils were included in the formulae.

Recipes

(a)

Mineral oil	5	Water	$42\frac{1}{2}$
Stearic acid	$1\frac{1}{2}$	Perfume oil	$\frac{1}{8}$
Cetyl alcohol	$\frac{1}{4}$		

(b)

Mineral oil	10	Glycerine	1
Cetyl alcohol	$\frac{1}{2}$	Water	39
Lanolin	$\frac{1}{2}$	Perfume oil	$\frac{1}{8}$

(c)

Mineral oil	$12\frac{1}{2}$	Cetyl alcohol	$\frac{1}{2}$
Ozokerite	$\frac{1}{2}$	Water	31
Paraffin wax	1	Perfume oil	$\frac{1}{8}$

(d) For oily or greasy skin

Triethanolamine lauryl sulphate	$2\frac{1}{2}$	Water	$47\frac{1}{2}$
		Perfume oil	$\frac{1}{8}$

Method To prepare *(a)*, *(b)* and *(c)* heat all the items except the water. When well blended add the water and the perfume oil. Stir until thoroughly mixed and cool. For *(d)*, mix by warming and stirring. The solution is then bottled.

(e)

Mineral oil	5	Triethanolamine	$\frac{3}{4}$
Cetyl alcohol	$\frac{1}{4}$	Water	$42\frac{1}{4}$
Stearic acid	$1\frac{1}{2}$	Perfume oil	$\frac{1}{8}$

Method Heat the mineral oil, cetyl alcohol and stearic acid until mixed, then dissolve the triethanolamine in the water and add this solution to the mixture, stirring continuously. As it cools add your chosen perfume oil. Thinner or thicker lotions may be made by increasing or reducing the quantity of water in the formula.

(f)

Diglycol laurate	7	Water	23
Liquid paraffin	20	Perfume oil	$\frac{1}{8}$

Method Mix the diglycol laurate with the liquid paraffin by shaking it vigorously in a closed container. Then add the water and perfume oil, stirring well.

(g)

Mineral oil	15	Glyceryl monostearate	$\frac{1}{4}$
Cetyl alcohol	$\frac{3}{4}$	Water	$33\frac{1}{2}$
Sodium lauryl sulphate	$\frac{1}{2}$	Perfume oil	$\frac{1}{8}$

Method Warm all the ingredients together and mix well, except the water. When blended, add the water and perfume oil, stirring continuously until cool.

(h)

Borax	1	Alcohol	20
Witchhazel	10	Water	69

Method Dissolve the borax in the water by heating it, then cool. Add the alcohol first, stirring well, and then the witchhazel. Make sure the whole mixture is well blended. If

necessary, filter the lotion through a piece of fine muslin or a
filter paper.

(i)

Glycerine	2	Water	97
Triethanolamine		Perfume oil	$\frac{1}{8}$
lauryl sulphate	1		

Method Warm the glycerine and dissolve the triethanolamine lauryl sulphate in it, then add the water and perfume
oil, stirring continuously.
Use This mixture may be used for cleansing tissues. Place a
small quantity on each tissue and seal the pads in airtight
containers or sachets.

(j)

| Boiling water | Enough to infuse the camomile and produce a tisane or tea | Camomile flower heads (dried) | 1 |

Method Allow to cool and use as a skin cleanser. It is
simplest to put the flower heads in a small muslin bag and
steep in a pint of boiling water. If necessary, strain the
infusion.

(k)

| Benzoin | A few drops | Water | As desired |

(l) For oily or greasy skin

| Propylene glycol | 5 | Triethanolamine lauryl | |
| Water | $42\frac{1}{2}$ | sulphate | $2\frac{1}{2}$ |

33

Method   Mix the propylene glycol and the triethanolamine lauryl sulphate together. Add the water and stir well, until properly blended.

Preserving   The same preservatives can be used as for cold creams. Otherwise keep the products in a refrigerator.

Glycerine and lemon lotion

Fresh lemon juice	5	Lemon or citral oil	$\frac{1}{8}$
Glycerine	5	Water	$38\frac{1}{2}$
Pectin	$1\frac{1}{2}$		

Method   Heat and mix together the glycerine, pectin, and water. Then cool and add the lemon juice and lemon or citral oil. The mixture may be filtered through muslin or filter paper before bottling. Keep in the refrigerator.

Herbal solution

Herbs	1

Take the selected herb, such as camomile, peppermint, rosemary or sage, and put it in a bowl. Pour two pints of boiling water over it to form a hot solution.
Use   Put the bowl of herbal solution on a table and place your face a foot above it, so that the steam rises directly on to your skin. Cover your head with a towel to stop the vapour escaping. Steam the skin for five minutes. Then remove the towel and splash cool water on to the skin to close the pores. Wipe gently to clean.

34

Softening and moisturizing creams and lotions

These are often termed night creams or emollients or moisturizing and nourishing creams and lotions. They tend to be heavier than cold or cleansing preparations. All-purpose creams can also be used for a similar purpose, though they can do different jobs for different people with varying types of skin, serving emollient, cleansing and foundation needs as the occasion arises.

(a)

Beeswax	4	Glyceryl monostearate	1
Petroleum jelly	$7\frac{1}{2}$	Borax	$\frac{1}{4}$
Mineral oil	13	Water	$17\frac{1}{2}$
Lanolin	$6\frac{3}{4}$	Perfume oil	$\frac{1}{8}$

(b)

Lanolin	$1\frac{1}{2}$	Sorbitol syrup	$1\frac{1}{2}$
Mineral oil	$1\frac{1}{2}$	Glycerine	$1\frac{1}{2}$
Petroleum jelly	$1\frac{1}{2}$	Water	35
Beeswax	$7\frac{1}{2}$	Perfume oil	$\frac{1}{8}$

(c)

Lanolin	1	Glycerine	$2\frac{1}{2}$
Cetyl alcohol	1	Glyceryl monostearate	7
Mineral oil	4	Water	28
Spermaceti	$2\frac{1}{2}$	Perfume oil	$\frac{1}{8}$
Almond oil	4		

(d)

Peanut or groundnut oil	$7\frac{1}{2}$	Beeswax	$2\frac{1}{2}$
Mineral oil	10	Borax	$\frac{1}{8}$
Petroleum jelly	15	Water	50
Lanolin	$2\frac{1}{2}$	Perfume oil	$\frac{1}{8}$

Reducing the amount of water makes a thicker cream.

(e)

Beeswax	5	Apricot or peach kernel oil	13
Spermaceti	$2\frac{1}{2}$		
Mineral oil	15	Water	$14\frac{1}{4}$
Borax	$\frac{1}{4}$	Perfume oil	$\frac{1}{8}$

(f)

Mineral oil	5	Glycerine	$12\frac{1}{2}$
Lanolin	5	Titanium dioxide	1
Glyceryl monostearate	$12\frac{1}{2}$	Water	$44\frac{1}{4}$
Stearic acid	$12\frac{1}{2}$	Perfume oil	$\frac{1}{4}$
Sorbitol	$7\frac{1}{2}$		

(g) Liquid cream or lotion

Petroleum jelly	$2\frac{1}{2}$	Glycerine	$1\frac{1}{4}$
Mineral oil	$22\frac{1}{2}$	Magnesium sulphate	$\frac{1}{10}$
Paraffin wax	$\frac{1}{2}$	Water	$21\frac{1}{4}$
Lanolin	1	Perfume oil	$\frac{1}{8}$
Sorbitan sesquioleate	1		

These recipes for creams and lotions should be prepared as for cleansing creams, by heating the solid materials and oils, mixing them well, and then adding the other items and the water with the perfume. If the preservatives already mentioned are not employed, the cosmetics should be stored in a refrigerator.

Note Various other oils, such as maize oil, olive oil and safflower oil, as well as different waxes including ceresine and ozokerite, may be used as substitutes for those listed.

For the treatment of lines and wrinkles around the eyes formulae containing olive and castor oils and lanolin are useful.

Eye wrinkle remover

Olive oil	1	Isopropyl myristate	1
Castor oil	8		

Method Mix well and apply gently.

All-purpose creams

(a)

Mineral oil	9	Sorbitan sesquioleate	$\frac{3}{4}$
Lanolin	1	Glycerol	$2\frac{1}{2}$
Petroleum jelly	1	Magnesium sulphate	$\frac{1}{10}$
Ozokerite	$3\frac{1}{2}$	Water	$30\frac{1}{2}$
Paraffin wax	$1\frac{1}{2}$	Perfume oil	$\frac{1}{8}$

(b)

Wool alcohol (wool fat distillate)	$12\frac{1}{2}$	Glycerine	25
		Magnesium sulphate	$3\frac{1}{2}$
Microcrystalline wax	30	Water	299
Mineral oil	105	Perfume oil	$\frac{1}{2}$
Petroleum jelly	25		

(c)

Wool alcohol	30	Liquid paraffin	300
Hard paraffin wax	120	Water	500
Soft white paraffin wax	50	Perfume oil	1

Method Preparation of these recipes is similar to other cosmetic creams. The solids and oils should be blended by heating and the water added slowly, stirring continuously. The chosen perfume oil is added with the water.

Hand creams and lotions

(a)

Rosewater	10	Honey	$\frac{3}{8}$
Glycerine	4	Perfume oil	$\frac{1}{16}$
White vinegar	$\frac{1}{8}$		

Method Mix ingredients well together and keep in a bottle.

(b)

Glycerine	$12\frac{1}{2}$	Rosewater	$37\frac{1}{2}$

Method Mix well and bottle.

(c)

Glycerine	5	Water	$43\frac{3}{4}$
Gum tragacanth	1	Perfume oil	$\frac{1}{8}$
Titanium dioxide	$\frac{1}{10}$		

Method Soak the tragacanth in the glycerine and water for twenty-four hours, put in a pan and heat to 158°F (70°C), stirring well. Allow the mixture to cool for forty-eight hours, then add the titanium dioxide and perfume and blend thoroughly.

(d)

Irish moss	$1\frac{1}{8}$	Water	$41\frac{1}{4}$
Alcohol	5	Perfume oil	$\frac{1}{8}$
Glycerine	$2\frac{1}{2}$		

Method Soak the Irish moss and the glycerine in the water for twenty-four hours. Then heat to 140°F (60°C) and leave to stand for forty-eight hours. Stir in the remaining items, blending thoroughly.

(e)

Quince seed	$\frac{1}{2}$	Cetyl alcohol	$\frac{1}{4}$
Karaya gum	$\frac{1}{6}$	Lanolin	$\frac{1}{2}$
Stearic acid	$\frac{3}{4}$	Water	49
Potassium hydroxide	$\frac{1}{8}$	Perfume oil	$\frac{1}{8}$
Glycerine	7		

Method Soak the karaya gum separately in some of the water and when it has formed a mucilage, or gluey mixture, stir it into the rest of the mixture, which should meanwhile have been well blended from the rest of the ingredients in the formula.

(f)

Paraffin wax	13	Perfume oil	$\frac{1}{8}$
Petroleum jelly	37		

(g)

Lanolin	$4\frac{1}{2}$	Paraffin wax	$9\frac{1}{4}$
Ceresine	9	Petroleum jelly	25
Amber resin	$2\frac{1}{4}$	Perfume oil	$\frac{1}{8}$

(h)

Paraffin wax	12	Camphor	$\frac{1}{10}$
Petroleum jelly	50	Zinc oxide	$\frac{1}{10}$
Birch tar oil	$\frac{1}{60}$	Eucalyptus oil	1
Benzoin	$\frac{1}{60}$	Methyl salicylate	$\frac{1}{5}$
Marshmallow leaf juice	$\frac{1}{15}$	Amber resin	4
Thyme oil	$\frac{1}{5}$	Paraffin wax	12
Citronella oil	$\frac{1}{10}$	Petroleum jelly	50

A thinner preparation may be made by decreasing the quantity of petroleum jelly.

(i) Camphor Ice

Paraffin wax	20	Camphor	10
White petroleum jelly	70		

The hardness may be varied by altering the ratio between the white petroleum jelly and the paraffin wax, or by increasing the camphor content to 15 ounces.

Note Recipes *(f)*, *(g)*, *(h)*, and *(i)* are for hard-block hand pomades, ie stiffer preparations.

(j)

Alcohol	5	Glycerol	5
Cetyl alcohol	2	Water	85
Wool alcohol	$2\frac{1}{2}$	Perfume oil	$\frac{1}{8}$

40

Method Hand creams and lotions should be prepared in a similar manner to other skin creams by heating and blending the solids and oils first and then adding the water, perfume and any other ingredients, if appropriate, stirring continuously, to form a good mixture.

(k) Elderberry hand ointment
Take a jar of petroleum jelly, heat it until the material is liquid and then stir in as many elderberry flowers as possible. Continue adding until no more can be absorbed, stirring continuously. Simmer gently for about fifty minutes. Then remove from the stove, pour through a sieve or muslin and into jars. Leave to cool.

Tonics and fresheners

These can be used as toning lotions after cleansing, to remove traces of grease or soap, and to give the skin a clean, fresh feeling. Skin foods are used to preserve the skin and to alleviate dry skin conditions.

Astringents

(a)

Glycerine	$2\frac{1}{2}$	Potassium aluminium	
Rosewater	25	sulphate	$\frac{1}{2}$
Zinc sulphate	$\frac{1}{8}$	Water	$21\frac{3}{4}$

(b)

Rosewater	$28\frac{1}{2}$	Zinc phenolsulphonate	1
Zinc sulphate	$\frac{1}{2}$	Water	20

(c)

Glycerine	3	Potassium aluminium	
Orange flower water	17½	sulphate	2
Rosewater	17½		

Method To prepare these three lotions, dissolve the aluminium or zinc salts in the water by heating and stirring gently. Then cool the solution and add the scented water(s). The lotion can be filtered through muslin or filter paper.

(d)

Glycerine	3	Alcohol	15
Witchhazel	30	Rosewater	52

Method Add the alcohol to the glycerine, stir well and then add the other ingredients.

(e)

A quick astringent treatment can be carried out by using a portion of cut cucumber dipped in fresh lemon juice and rubbed gently over the skin. Lime juice is also suitable.

(f)

Glycerine	25	Zinc sulphate	1
Alcohol	100	Witchhazel	125
Menthol	½	Sorbitol	1
Camphor	½	Rosewater or water	240
Potassium alum	6	Perfume oil	½

Method Mix the perfume oil with the sorbitol, then add part of the rosewater or water. Dissolve the potassium alum and the zinc sulphate in the remaining water and add to the first mixture. Then dissolve the menthol and camphor in the alcohol and add this solution too. The whole mixture should then be well stirred and thoroughly blended.

Soothing lotion

Calamine powder	75	Resorcin	10
Glycerine	75	Cetrimide	$2\frac{1}{2}$
Zinc oxide	25	Alcohol	25
Bentonite	10	Water	$252\frac{1}{2}$
Flowers of sulphur	15		

Method   Sieve the bentonite, calamine and zinc powders. Then mix it to a smooth paste with some of the glycerine, adding this drop by drop. Now dissolve the cetrimide in the rest of the glycerine, adding some of the water to this mixture. Then mix the sulphur and the resorcin with the alcohol. Combine all these three mixtures, adding the rest of the water, to form one well-blended lotion.

Lotion for spotty faces

Sodium bicarbonate	5	Alcohol	$12\frac{1}{2}$
Borax	10	Glycerine	50
Menthol	$\frac{1}{10}$	Water	$422\frac{1}{4}$
Thymol	$\frac{1}{10}$	Purified talc or	
Methyl salicylate	$\frac{1}{10}$	kiesulguhr	As required

Method   Dissolve the sodium bicarbonate and borax in the water. Then add the glycerine and mix well. Now dissolve the menthol, thymol, and methyl salicylate in the alcohol.

Combine these two solutions. Place a little purified talc or kiesulguhr in a bowl and add small amounts of the mixture steadily, stirring well all the time. Continue until finished, replenishing the purified talc as required. The aim is to thicken the mixture with enough purified talc to form a spreading lotion.

Skin tonics

(a)

Glycerine	5	Zinc phenolsulphonate	$\frac{1}{2}$
Camphor	$\frac{1}{2}$	Rosewater	20
Alcohol	5	Water	25

(b)

Menthol	$\frac{1}{20}$	Potassium aluminium	
Orange flower water	15	sulphate	$\frac{1}{4}$
Alcohol	10	Water	$9\frac{3}{4}$
Rosewater	15		

(c)

Alcohol	5	Any herbal oil, such as
Borax	1	thyme, basil, dill or
Rosewater	20	fennel to give a pleasant
Water	24	odour (optional)

Note In making the above preparations the salts should first be dissolved in the water and the solids in the alcohol, and the other ingredients then added, stirring well. Combine all the mixtures to form one well-blended lotion.

Honey and almond cream

Almond oil	25	Glycerine	25
Beeswax	5	Water	325
Spermaceti	10	Perfume (almond	
Borax	1½	essence)	1–2
Soap powder	12½		

Method   Warm the almond oil, beeswax and spermaceti. Do the same with the other ingredients and add the latter to the former, stirring well. Cool and put in a jar.

Glycerine jelly

Glycerine	60	Boric acid crystals	7½
Alcohol	60	Water	367½
Gum tragacanth	5	Perfume oil	¾

Method   Mix the gum tragacanth with the alcohol and then add the glycerine and perfume oil. Now dissolve the boric acid in the water, warming as necessary, and then mix with the other ingredients, stirring continuously.

Skin foods

(a) For greasy skins

2 tomatoes, puréed	2 teaspoonfuls fresh lemon juice

Mix well together and apply to greasy or oily skin areas. After half-an-hour rinse off.

(b)

Take a small muslin bag and half fill it with oatmeal or porridge oats. Place it in warm water and use to sponge the skin.

(c)

Wheatgerm meal	2	Natural yogurt	2

Mix well, apply, leave for a quarter of an hour and rinse off.

(d)

Honey	2	2 egg whites	
Fresh lemon juice	$\frac{1}{2}$		

Mix well together, leave on your skin for twenty minutes and rinse off.

(e) For skin nourishment

Sunflower seed oil	12	Wheatgerm oil	$\frac{3}{4}$
Witchhazel	6	Perfume oil (any)	$\frac{1}{16}$
Lanolin	$3\frac{1}{4}$		

Method Melt the lanolin in a pot, then add the sunflower seed oil. Allow to cool slightly and mix in the witchhazel, followed by the wheatgerm oil. Then add the perfume oil.

(f)

Mineral oil	38	Lanolin	2
Petroleum jelly	8	Borax	1
White beeswax	15	Water	35
Paraffin wax	1	Perfume oil (if desired)	$\frac{1}{4}$

46

Method Dissolve the borax in the water. Warm the other ingredients and mix them well together. Now add the water and borax solution to the second mixture, stirring all the time, and blend satisfactorily.

For dry skins

(g)

Honey	$2\frac{1}{2}$	2 egg yolks

Mix well and leave on the skin for quarter of an hour, then rinse with cool water.

(h)

Olive oil	2	2 egg yolks

Mix well and leave on the skin for twenty minutes, then rinse in luke-warm water.

(i)

Fruits such as banana, peach, papaya or avocado may be puréed and applied to the skin for twenty minutes, then rinsed off with warm water.

Smoothing and boosting

(j)

Honey	2	Thin cream	2

Mix well and apply for three minutes to the skin, then rinse off.

(k)

Apricots, fresh or dried fruits, which have been well soaked in water, may be puréed and used as a skin smoother.

Face packs and masks

These are intended to improve the condition of the skin by removing surface debris and helping circulation. Take care not to put face packs or masks on the area of the eyes.

(a) General-purpose

Fuller's earth	As required	Honey	$\frac{1}{4}$
Milk	2		

Method Mix the milk and honey and then add enough Fuller's earth to produce a face pack to your liking.

(b)

Soak oatmeal or porridge oats in boiling milk and apply to your face when nearly cool. Wash off with warm water and rinse.

(c)

Kaolin	50	Glyceryl monostearate	25
Flowers of sulphur	1	Glycerine	15
Bentonite	50	Menthol	$\frac{1}{2}$
Zinc oxide	50	Alcohol	50
Cetrimide	1	Water	251
Gum acacia	$2\frac{1}{2}$	Perfume oil (if desired)	$\frac{1}{2}$

Method Mix the water and glycerine and add the gum acacia and the glyceryl monostearate, heating them to dissolve them. Mix up the other ingredients, sieve, and add to the mixture already prepared. Stir until smooth and ready for use.

(d)

Microcrystalline wax	$6\frac{1}{2}$	Mineral oil	10
Paraffin wax	30	Bentonite	$\frac{3}{4}$
Cetyl alcohol	$2\frac{1}{2}$	Isopropyl alcohol	$\frac{1}{4}$

Method Mix the solids together by heating and then add the other ingredients, blending well together.

(e)

White gelatine	$1\frac{1}{8}$	Zinc oxide	$1\frac{1}{4}$
Gum tragacanth	1	Water	40
Glycerine	$1\frac{1}{4}$	Honey	$4\frac{1}{2}$

Method Dissolve the gum tragacanth in the water by warming, then add the other ingredients and mix well.

(f)

Gelatine	5	Titanium oxide	1
Camphor	$\frac{1}{4}$	Alcohol	A little to dissolve
Zinc oxide	$1\frac{1}{2}$		the camphor
Kaolin	$2\frac{1}{2}$	Water	25

Method Dissolve the camphor in a little alcohol, warm the water, add the other ingredients and stir well.

Note Face packs *(e)* and *(f)* should be applied warm to the skin. This means heating them before use, if they have been made up previously and left to cool.

(g)

Casein	10	Glycerine	$2\frac{1}{2}$
Borax	$\frac{1}{4}$	Water	50

Method Dissolve the borax in the water. Mix the casein with the glycerine and then add to the water, using heat.

(h) For dry skin

Kaolin	40	Olive oil	$2\frac{1}{2}$
Starch	5	Water	Enough to produce
Cold cream	10		desired consistency
Cetyl alcohol	1		of pack or mask

Method Melt the cold cream and the cetyl alcohol in some warm water. Then add the olive oil, kaolin and starch, mixing well and using more water to bring the mixture to the desired consistency.

(i) For greasy skin

Kaolin	40	Gum tragacanth	$\frac{1}{2}$
Magnesium carbonate	$7\frac{1}{2}$	Water	As required
Starch	$2\frac{1}{2}$		

Method Dissolve the magnesium carbonate and gum tragacanth in some hot water, then add the other ingredients with enough extra water to get a satisfactory mixture.

Eye lotions

These help to relieve strain and irritation and keep the eyes beautiful.

(a)

Boric acid crystals	1	Distilled water	$98\frac{3}{4}$
Zinc sulphate	$\frac{1}{5}$		

(b)

Sodium borate	$\frac{1}{2}$	Sodium chloride	$\frac{1}{2}$
Glycerine	2	Distilled water	92
Witchhazel	5		

(c)

Boric acid crystals	2	Witchhazel (distilled)	20
Zinc sulphate	$\frac{1}{10}$	Distilled water	$173\frac{1}{2}$
Glycerine	4		

Method The salts should be dissolved in the water by warming and stirring. Any other ingredients should then be added, blending the mixture well.

Cosmetic eye drops

This lotion, which is also antiseptic, imparts an attractive blue tint to the whites of the eyes.

Sodium chloride		Methylene blue	$\frac{1}{100}$
(common salt)	$4\frac{1}{2}$	Distilled water	$495\frac{1}{4}$

Method Dissolve the sodium chloride in the water and add drops of methylene blue. Stir well.

For swollen or puffy eyes, dried mint infused with boiling water (mint tea) or milk are often helpful.

Suntan oils and lotions

Heliotherapy or sunbathing was known for centuries to have beneficial effects on the skin as well as to combat fatigue and apathy. Today a suntan is fashionable and desirable, but very painful results can come from overexposure to the sun's rays.

Sunburn preparations should be stable to heat, light and perspiration, be non-irritant and non-toxic, and should not be rapidly absorbed by the skin.

Sunscreening agents are available from various companies (see the list of suppliers) and can be used in the recipes here:

Suntan cream paste

Vaseline	$18\frac{1}{4}$	Calcium stearate	5
Mineral oil	$7\frac{1}{2}$	Kaolin	15
Sesame oil	1	Sunscreening agent	$2\frac{1}{2}$
Stearyl alcohol	$1\frac{3}{4}$		

Method Mix by heating as you would for cold and other creams. The sunscreening agent is usually dissolved in the oil, but if the manufacturer says it is susceptible to high temperatures it may be stirred into the mixture as it cools.

Suntan oils

(a)

Sesame oil	$12\frac{1}{2}$	Sunscreening agent	$2\frac{1}{2}$
Mineral oil	25	Perfume oil (if desired)	$\frac{1}{8}$
Isopropyl myristate	$12\frac{1}{2}$	Colour	As required

Olive oil	5	Sunscreening agent	$2\frac{1}{4}$
Sesame oil	20	Perfume oil (if desired)	$\frac{1}{8}$
Mineral oil	$23\frac{3}{4}$	Colour	As required

Method   Stir the ingredients well together so that they are thoroughly blended.

Suntan lotion

Glycerine	1	Alcohol	5
Methyl cellulose	$\frac{1}{4}$	Sunscreening agent	2
Water	$40\frac{1}{4}$		

Method   Mix well until properly blended.

Creams

(a) Non-greasy

Lanolin	1	Sodium hydroxide	$\frac{1}{20}$
Glycerine	$2\frac{1}{2}$	Water	$38\frac{1}{4}$
Stearic acid	$7\frac{1}{2}$	Sunscreening agent	$2\frac{1}{4}$
Cetyl alcohol	$\frac{1}{4}$	Perfume and colour	
Potassium hydroxide	$\frac{1}{4}$		As desired

Method   Mix together by heating the stearic acid, the cetyl alcohol and the lanolin. In a separate container, do the same with the potassium and sodium hydroxides, the glycerine and the water. Add this when well mixed to the first mixture and stir thoroughly, putting in the sunscreening agent as the mixture cools, with perfume oil and colour if desired.

(b) Greasy

Sesame oil	5	Water	28
Glycerine	3½	Sunscreening agent	2½
Mineral oil	5	Perfume and colour	
Glyceryl monostearate	8		As desired
Cetyl alcohol	½		

Method Mix together the glyceryl monostearate, the cetyl alcohol and the sesame and mineral oils. In a separate pan, do the same with the other ingredients, heating and adding to the first lot. Stir continuously and add the sunscreening agent during cooling, with perfume and colour if desired.

Sunburn relievers

Calamine lotions

(a)

Calamine	10	Water	37½
Glycerine	2½		

Method Mix well and shake before application. A little antiseptic may be added to this lotion.

(b)

Calamine	15	Alcohol	10
Camphor	1	Glycerine	10
Zinc oxide	5	Rose or lime water	59

Method Mix well and shake before using. It is best to combine the calamine and zinc oxide first as a smooth paste with the glycerine, and then add enough rose or lime water to make a cream. Now dissolve the camphor in the alcohol, add this solution and top up with the rest of the water.

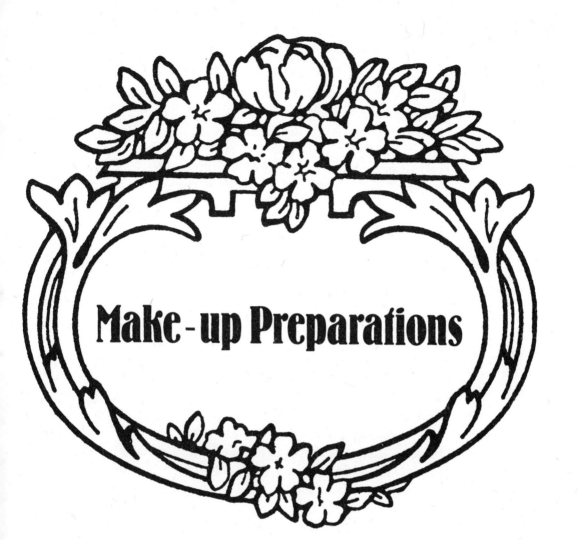

Make-up Preparations

Foundations are the basis of daily make-up. Vanishing creams are the traditional types, but today plain or coloured foundations, highlight sticks and creams and other products can be made to suit individual preferences. Preservatives may be added to all these cosmetics. When mixing up vanishing creams it is important to make the first emulsion while hot, and to get good consistency, sheen and texture, the cream should be well stirred during and just after cooling.

Traditional vanishing creams

(a)

Glycerine	4	Water	38
Stearic acid	$7\frac{1}{2}$	Perfume oil	$\frac{1}{8}$
Potassium hydroxide	$\frac{1}{4}$		

Method Heat the stearic acid to 167°F (75°C). Then dissolve the potassium hydroxide and the glycerine in the water at the same temperature, adding this mixture to the stearic acid. Stir continuously, add the perfume and cool, allowing the mixture to stand for one to two days.

(b)

Glycerine	4	Triethanolamine	$\frac{5}{8}$
Stearic acid	10	Water	35
Cetyl alcohol	$\frac{1}{4}$	Perfume oil	$\frac{1}{8}$
Sodium hydroxide	$\frac{1}{3}$		

Method Heat the stearic acid and the cetyl alcohol until well mixed. Then dissolve the triethanolamine and the sodium hydroxide in the glycerine and water, warming to 167°F (75°C). Now add this to the first mixture, stirring continuously. Finally add the perfume oil. Allow the mixture to cool and stand for one to two days.

(c)

Stearic acid	$7\frac{1}{2}$	Potassium hydroxide	$\frac{3}{8}$
Cetyl alcohol	$\frac{1}{4}$	Water	$39\frac{1}{4}$
Glycerol	$2\frac{1}{2}$	Perfume oil	$\frac{1}{8}$

Method   Heat the stearic acid and the cetyl alcohol, mix well, then add the potassium hydroxide in the glycerol and water and combine the two mixtures. Stir continuously, cool and leave to stand for two days.

(d)

Stearic acid	45	Glycerine	40
Cetyl alcohol	$2\frac{1}{2}$	Potassium hydroxide	5
Soap powder (pure soap curd)	$2\frac{1}{2}$	Water	360
		Perfume	$\frac{1}{2}$ to $\frac{3}{4}$

Method   Heat the stearic acid and the cetyl alcohol in one pan and the other ingredients, except the perfume oil, in another. Then add the latter to the former, stirring continuously. Allow to cool and add the essential perfume oil when lukewarm.

(e)

Mineral oil	20	Glycerine	60
Cetyl alcohol	15	Water	345
Glyceryl monostearate	60	Perfume oil	$\frac{1}{2}$

Method Heat the mineral oil, the cetyl alcohol and the glyceryl monostearate in one container and the other items, except the perfume oil, in another, mixing well. Then add the latter to the former, stirring continuously, and cool. Add the perfume oil when lukewarm.

(f) For dry, flaky skin

Lanolin	5	Glycerine	25
Mineral oil	50	Triethanolamine	$2\frac{1}{2}$
Stearic acid	$12\frac{1}{2}$	Water	390
Glyceryl monostearate	15	Perfume oil	$\frac{1}{2}$

Method Heat the lanolin, mineral oil, stearic acid and the glyceryl monostearate in one pan, and the rest of the items, except the perfume oil, in another. Then mix the latter with the former, stir well, and finally add the perfume oil when lukewarm.

Foundations

Foundation creams should look nice, spread well, and give even coverage without dragging or rolling. Where powder is used the foundation must make it cling well. The film produced by foundations should look matt.

(a)

Stearic acid	9	Sodium hydroxide	$\frac{1}{10}$
Cetyl alcohol	$\frac{1}{4}$	Water	31
Glycerine	9	Perfume oil	$\frac{1}{8}$
Potassium hydroxide	$\frac{1}{4}$		

Method Heat the stearic acid and cetyl alcohol, and mix

well. Then heat the other ingredients and add them to the first mixture. Stir continuously and when lukewarm add the perfume oil. Cool and leave to stand for a day or two.

(b)

Petroleum jelly	$42\frac{1}{2}$	Perfume oil	$\frac{1}{8}$
Zinc oxide	$7\frac{1}{2}$		

Method   Mix the zinc oxide with the petroleum jelly by heating and stirring, then cool, adding perfume oil. Water may be added if you like, or if you find it necessary in mixing.

(c)

Olive oil	125	Kaolin	110
Mineral oil	110	Isopropyl palmitate	15
Ozokerite	$2\frac{1}{4}$	Titanium dioxide	$102\frac{3}{4}$
Carnauba wax	$13\frac{3}{4}$	Perfume oil	1
Beeswax	20		

Method   Mix together by heating and stirring the olive and mineral oils, and the three waxes. Then add the other ingredients and blend well. Finally add the perfume while cooling and stand for a day or two.

(d) Stick-type

Petroleum jelly	50	Isopropyl myristate	$37\frac{1}{2}$
Castor oil	150	Titanium dioxide	50
Ozokerite	10	Perfume oil	$\frac{1}{4}$
Candelilla wax	20		

Method   Heat the petroleum jelly and the oil and waxes to blend them well. Then sieve the titanium dioxide and mix to a smooth paste with the isopropyl myristate, adding to the other mixture. Stir well and pour into suitable containers, after adding perfume oil.

(e) Moisturizing foundation

Lanolin	$17\frac{1}{2}$	Propylene glycol	30
Stearic acid	10	Glycerine	20
Isopropyl myristate	10	Titanium dioxide	25
Glyceryl monostearate	$7\frac{1}{2}$	Talc	25
Cetyl alcohol	$7\frac{1}{2}$	Water	$342\frac{1}{2}$
Triethanolamine	5	Perfume oil	$\frac{1}{2}$

Method Mix together by heating and stirring the lanolin, stearic acid and the isopropyl myristate, glyceryl monostearate and the cetyl alcohol. Heat the triethanolamine and water and add to the mixture. Then mix the titanium dioxide with the glycerine and propylene glycol to form a paste. While stirring add this paste to the main mixture. Continue stirring and when well blended allow to cool, adding the perfume oil during this process.

Coloured foundations

To produce coloured foundations, pigments are added in appropriate amounts to the mixtures. They should be made into a paste with some of the water or glycerine from the recipe. Only very small quantities are necessary. For examples, the following colours can be obtained with the procedure below. Only cosmetic grades of pigments should be used.

In 180 ounces of foundation cream use pigments in these quantities (also in ounces) to obtain the shades given:

Natural Red oxide $\frac{1}{4}$, yellow oxide $\frac{5}{8}$
Beige Red oxide $\frac{1}{5}$, yellow oxide $1\frac{1}{3}$, umber $\frac{1}{3}$
Deep beige Red oxide $\frac{1}{6}$, yellow oxide $1\frac{1}{2}$, umber $\frac{5}{8}$
Tan Red oxide $\frac{5}{8}$, yellow oxide $1\frac{1}{3}$, umber $\frac{5}{8}$

Face powders

Face powders have several functions – to hide skin blemishes, to prevent shine and give a matt or peach-like appearance, and to enhance general beauty. Good products cling perfectly to the skin, do not blow off easily and last for a reasonable time. They should also spread well and give a natural look. The ingredients of face powders are many and varied, including materials such as colloidal kaolin, talc, precipitated chalk, rice starch, zinc oxide, magnesium carbonate, magnesium and zinc stearates, powdered silica and silicates, powdered silk, pigments and perfumes.

Here are some general recipes for making face powders:

(a) Light-type powder

Talc	40	Zinc stearate	$2\frac{1}{2}$
Rice starch	5	Perfume oil and	
Zinc oxide	$2\frac{1}{2}$	colour	As desired

(b) Opaque matt finish

Talc	15	Zinc stearate	3
Precipitated chalk	20	Perfume and	
Zinc oxide	12	colour	As desired

Note Precipitated chalk may be substituted for the starch.

61

General

(c)

Talc	30	Zinc stearate	2½
Kaolin	10	Perfume oil and	
Zinc oxide	7½	colour	As desired

(d)

Talc	32½	Zinc stearate	2½
Precipitated chalk	5	Perfume oil and	
Zinc oxide	10	colour	As desired

Medium

(e)

Talc	25	Zinc stearate	2½
Rice starch	7½	Perfume oil and	
Precipitated chalk	7½	colour	As desired
Zinc oxide	7½		

(f)

Kaolin	8	Zinc oxide	8
Precipitated chalk	9	Zinc stearate	2½
Rice starch	4	Perfume oil and	
Talc	18½	colour	As desired

Heavy

(g)

Talc	100	Zinc oxide	75
Kaolin	100	Perfume oils and	
Precipitated chalk	200	colour	As desired
Magnesium stearate	25		

62

(h)

Kaolin	125	Zinc oxide	75
Precipitated chalk	75	Magnesium stearate	25
Talc	175	Perfume oils and	
Titanium dioxide	25	colour	As desired

Preparation   Mixing and sifting are important for making up powders. A 120-mesh sieve is excellent. It is best to brush the materials twice through the sieve. A cardboard ring to raise the top part of the sieve above the mesh ensures that no materials are lost. Small mixers or milling machines are available for preparing powders and any device that will blend the different ingredients well together can be used.

Powder preparation consists of mixing together the main ingredients and then adding the perfume oils and colours bit by bit, or by spraying to ensure an even distribution throughout the mixture. After this has been done, the powder is then sieved as described above.

Colours   Specially prepared colours for face powders are available from manufacturers. It is generally considered that Naturelle is best for blondes and Rachel for brunettes. Peach is also suitable for fair skins. Naturelle should always have a slightly bluish tint. To tone down a florid complexion a pale bluish-green tinted powder is helpful.

Perfumes   Face powders may be scented by using mixtures of perfume or essential oils (see Chapter 6) or by adding ready-made scents in any quantity desired.

The amounts of colours and perfumes added to recipes can be selected individually according to taste, but take care not to use too much of these ingredients and to build up the colour and scent by gradual addition.

Fatty powder for rough or dry skin

Petroleum jelly	45	Talc	500
White beeswax	20	Water	250
Stearine	10	Perfume oils and	
Glyceryl monostearate	$37\frac{1}{2}$	colour	As desired

Method Melt the fatty materials and mix well together. Then add the water while stirring continuously, and when an emulsion has formed add the talc. Continue mixing until well blended. Then knead the mixture, allow it to dry, rub it into a powder, add the perfume oils and colour and pass twice through a sieve.

Compact powders are face powders to which binding agents such as soap, oils, gums or other materials are added in small amounts to make the powder stick together, so that it can be pressed into a compact case. The easiest binders to employ are mineral oil, lanolin, isopropyl myristate, tragacanth, karaya and arabic gums, glyceryl monostearate or triethanolamine. Generally, only one to two per cent of binder is needed to make face powders suitable for compacting.

Cake make-up – Here the normal constituents of a face powder mixture are combined with both oil and water to form a paste-like substance similar to a powder cream. This is then dried, ground, and compressed into a cake. Cake powder make-up is applied wet so that it dries on the skin.

Rouge

Rouges may be made in liquid, cream, paste and powder forms.

Liquid

Mineral oil	6	Triethanolamine	2
Acetylated monoglyceride (liquid)	6	Water	26
		Perfume oil	$\frac{1}{16}$
Isopropyl myristate	6	Colour or pigments	1
Oleic acid	4	Bromo acid	$\frac{1}{20}$

Method Mix together the mineral oil, acetylated monogly-ceride and isopropyl myristate. Grind up the pigments, add them to the mixture and heat. At the same time place all the other ingredients, except the perfume oil, in another container, heat, then blend them gradually into the first mixture. Cool, stirring continuously, and adding in the perfume oil.

Cream

(a)

Petroleum jelly	7	Pigment or colour	As desired
Kaolin	3	Perfume oil	As desired

Method Grind the colour with the kaolin and stir this into the petroleum jelly. Mix well, using heat.

(b)

Beeswax	$2\frac{1}{2}$	Mineral oil	$3\frac{3}{4}$
Cetyl alcohol	$1\frac{1}{4}$	Colour	As desired
Stearic acid	$3\frac{1}{2}$	Perfume oil	As desired
Petroleum jelly	$38\frac{1}{2}$		

Method Mix the colour with the oil and fats, and then, using heat, blend all together to form a smooth cream.

(c)

Beeswax	7	Borax	$\frac{3}{8}$
Lanolin	$2\frac{1}{2}$	Water	22
Cocoa butter	$2\frac{1}{2}$	Perfume oil and	
Liquid paraffin	15	colour	As desired
Cetyl alcohol	$\frac{1}{2}$		

Method Mix the powdered colour with the fats and oils which should be melted, then dissolve the borax in the water, heating it, and mix all together well, stirring continuously. Finally cool, adding the perfume oil.

(d)

Glycerine	4	Water	$28\frac{1}{4}$
Stearic acid	$7\frac{1}{2}$	Colour	As desired
Potassium hydroxide	$\frac{1}{4}$	Perfume oil	As desired
Sodium hydroxide	$\frac{1}{12}$		

Method Prepare as for the other rouge creams.

Powder

Talc	41	Perfume oil	As desired
Titanium dioxide	$2\frac{1}{2}$	Binder, if a compact	
Colour	As desired	powder is wanted	

Method Mix together ingredients. The binder is made from mineral oil 1 part, sorbitan sesquioleate $\frac{3}{8}$ of a part, and water $2\frac{1}{4}$ parts; 5 ounces of this binder should be added.

Pastes

Pastes are made in the same manner with a small amount of petroleum jelly included.

66

Note Bromo acid (mentioned in the formula for liquid rouge) of red or orange tone gives a natural blushing effect. For colours or pigments for rouges see information on lipsticks, below.

Lipsticks

Lipsticks must colour the lips attractively and smoothly and be absolutely safe and non-toxic. Nor should the colour come off unreasonably in ordinary circumstances. Apart from a good degree of plasticity, a lipstick must have a pleasant taste and an agreeable odour.

The main parts of a lipstick formula consist of waxes, oils, bromo mixture or solution of staining dyestuff, blended with suitable materials, colours, flavours, and preservatives.

Here is a useful general-purpose mixture:

Castor oil	5	Eosol stearate	11
Beeswax	10	Cetyl alcohol	1
Ozokerite	3	Bromo acid	1
Lanolin	5	Colour and flavour	
Liquid paraffin	10		As desired

Method Dissolve the bromo acid in the eosol and put it aside. Mix the colours with some of the castor oil to form a paste. Blend these two mixtures well together. Heat and mix the other ingredients and add them to the first mixture. Stir continuously until the whole mass is thoroughly combined. The flavour can now be added with some perfume oil to give a mild but pleasant odour. The lipstick should be poured into suitably-shaped moulds, possibly old or ready-made lipstick containers, smeared inside with liquid paraffin to prevent it sticking to them when cold, and left to cool.

Ready-made colours for lipsticks can be bought from various firms. Shades available are usually basic (red, pink and orange); pastel (rose, peach) and blue, yellow and opalescent pastes.

Lip salve

(a)

Mineral oil	9	Spermaceti	6
Beeswax	5		

(b)

Lanolin	3	Paraffin wax	7
Petroleum jelly (white)	10		

Method Heat all the ingredients and blend them well together. Dyestuff can be added to produce rose or pink colouring.

Lip jelly

This produces a high gloss if applied over a lipstick.

(a)

Petroleum jelly	5	Lanolin	5

(b)

Castor oil	1	Lanolin	9

Method These recipes should be well mixed and can be tinted with dyestuff or colours and perfumed.

Mascara

This may be made in cake, liquid or cream form.

Cake mascara

(a)

Beeswax	3	Triethanolamine	$1\frac{1}{5}$
Carnauba wax	5	Colour	$2\frac{1}{2}$
Stearic acid	$2\frac{3}{4}$		

Method   The ingredients should be well mixed by heating and then allowed to cool.

(b)

Cocoa butter	$\frac{1}{2}$	Paraffin wax	$\frac{1}{2}$
Petroleum jelly (white)	$5\frac{1}{2}$	Colour	$4\frac{1}{2}$

Colour   Black is a popular colour for mascara but other shades are available. Lampblack is used, and there are ranges of carbon blacks and different hues of cosmetic grade made by various firms.

Liquid mascara

Alcohol	1	Water	$10\frac{1}{4}$
Gum tragacanth	$\frac{1}{20}$	Lampblack	1

Method   Prepare by dissolving the gum in the water by heating, then mix in the other ingredients and cool.

Cream mascara

(a)

Mucilage of quince		Sugar syrup (3 parts of sugar	
seeds	7	to 2 parts of water)	$2\frac{1}{3}$
Gum arabic	7	Colour	$4\frac{1}{2}$

Method Grind up the gum and the colouring and mix with the sugar syrup, then add to the mucilage (quince seeds soaked in a little water). A preservative may be incorporated.

(b)

Paraffin wax	$5\frac{1}{2}$	Mineral oil	$1\frac{1}{2}$
Carnauba wax	$6\frac{1}{2}$	Triethanolamine	$4\frac{3}{4}$
Microcrystalline wax	2	Colour	20
Stearic acid	$10\frac{1}{2}$	Water	49

Method Heat together the paraffin wax, microcrystalline wax, stearic acid and mineral oil and mix well. Then blend thoroughly with the colouring, stirring continuously until the mixture is quite smooth. Now add the carnauba wax and the triethanolamine which should have been heated separately before incorporation. Continue stirring until cool.

Eyeshadow

Cream

Petroleum jelly	12	Isopropyl myristate	33
Lanolin (liquid)	1	Perfume oil	$\frac{1}{16}$
Microcrystalline wax	2	Colour	$18\frac{1}{4}$
Beeswax	1		

Method Melt all the ingredients and mix them well together, pour into moulds and leave to get cold. The colours or pigments may be obtained from various firms.

Powder

| Talc | 4 | Titanium dioxide | $1\frac{5}{8}$ |
| Magnesium myristate | $4\frac{3}{8}$ | Colour pigments | As desired |

Method Mix the colour with some of the talc and sieve. Sieve the titanium dioxide separately and then mix all the ingredients together. Sieve again and blend well.

Eyebrow pencils

Beeswax	8	Butyl stearate	3
Lanolin	1	Mineral oil	5
Castor oil	$8\frac{1}{3}$	Perfume oil	$\frac{1}{4} - \frac{1}{8}$
Ozokerite	8	Colour	As desired

Method Heat all the items and mix well. Stir and strain through muslin cloth and then pour into moulds to give thin pencil shapes. Leave to get cold.

Eyeliner

Glycerine	5	Diethylene glycol	
Lanolin	$\frac{1}{2}$	monostearate	3
Magnesium aluminium		Sodium lauryl sulphate	1
silicate	$2\frac{1}{2}$	Water	76
Polyvinyl pyrrolidone	2	Colour	10

Method   Mix the magnesium aluminium silicate with water and dissolve the polyvinyl pyrrolidone in water also. Warm gently and add to the lanolin and the diethylene glycol monostearate, which should be already melted. Now mix the colouring with the glycerine and blend all these mixtures together. Stir well and add the sodium lauryl sulphate, dissolved in a little water, and the rest of the water. Work until a good cream is formed.

Removers

Eye make-up removers are made of mixtures of mineral oils with isopropyl myristate. The proportions are 3 parts of oil to 1 part of isopropyl myristate.

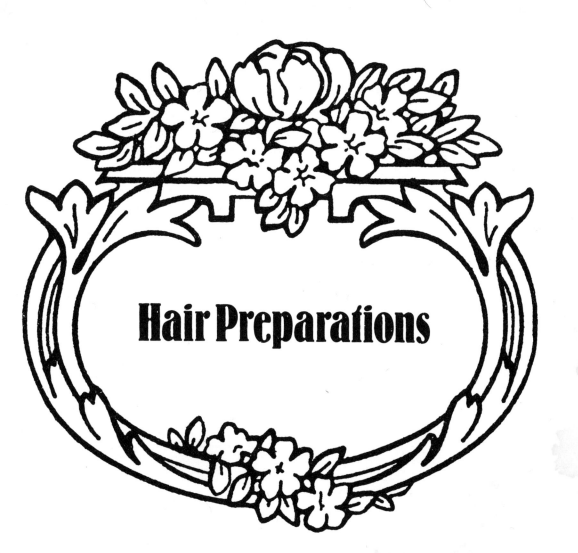

Hair Preparations

Hair is a precious possession and once lost can seldom be regained. Everyone should look after their hair. In practice, this means keeping it clean, free from infections and disease, and in good condition so that baldness, falling hair, dandruff, greying and other problems may be avoided or at least postponed.

The first job is to shampoo the hair properly. Good shampoos should remove dirt and other matter, leave no residue, and make the hair soft, lustrous and sweet-smelling.

Shampoos

These can be prepared in the form of powders, liquids or liquid creams, lotions, creams and jellies. Normally all shampoos are used with water, but in some cases it is desirable or necessary to use a dry powder shampoo.

Powders (to mix with water)

(a)

Sodium bicarbonate	5	Soap powder	3
Disodium phosphate	2	Perfume oil	A few drops as desired

(b)

Borax	15	Potassium carbonate	5
Henna powder	5	Soap powder	50
Sodium carbonate	25	Perfume oil	$\frac{1}{2}$

(c)

Powdered camomile flowers	5	Sodium carbonate	20
		Soap powder	50
Borax	25	Perfume oil	$\frac{1}{2}$

Method To prepare these three recipes mix all the ingredients together, then add the perfume oil, a few drops at a time, to ensure even distribution.

Note Shampoos containing soap powder should only be used in soft, pure, or distilled water; in hard water they are not very satisfactory. Rainwater is suitable if it is uncontaminated. However, a good final rinse with water containing a little lemon juice, vinegar, or citric or tartaric acid helps considerably. If the local water is hard, substitute sodium lauryl sulphate for soap powder. This can be bought as a white, free-flowing powder at different concentrations. For general use, a 45 per cent sodium lauryl sulphate is satisfactory.

Dry shampoos

(a)

Talc	40	Starch	15
Kieselguhr	45	Perfume oil A small amount	

(b)

Talc	25	Starch	70
Borax	5	Perfume oil A small amount	

Method Mix well together, with a small amount of perfume oil to scent it. Use dry, rubbing the powder through the hair and over the scalp. Leave for about ten minutes and then brush out thoroughly.

Liquids and liquid creams

These liquid shampoos are based on detergents, which are more suitable than soaps for all waters.

(a)

Triethanolamine lauryl sulphate	$22\frac{1}{2}$	Perfume oil	$\frac{1}{4}$
		Colour essence	As desired
Coconut monoethanolamide	1	Water	38

Method Mix together the triethanolamine lauryl sulphate and the coconut monoethanolamide, warming gently; then add the other ingredients, stirring thoroughly.

(b)

Monoethanolamine lauryl sulphate	7	Magnesium sulphate	$\frac{1}{4}$
		Propylene glycol monostearate	$\frac{5}{8}$
Coconut monoethanolamide	1	Perfume oil	As desired
Sodium hydroxide	$\frac{1}{10}$	Water	39
Stearic acid	$\frac{3}{4}$	Colour essence	As desired

Method Mix together, with slow heat, the monoethanolamine lauryl sulphate, the coconut monoethanolamide and the stearic acid, then add the water in which has been dissolved the magnesium sulphate, followed by the sodium hydroxide and propylene glycol monostearate. Finally add the remaining ingredients. Stir thoroughly to blend.

The ingredients used are shampoo bases of sulphonated fatty alcohols, obtained from coconut or palm kernel oils.

Often herb oils, egg, lanolin, beer and other items are added to shampoos to give particular formulae.

Egg shampoo

Ethylene glycol		Egg powder or dried	
monostearate	3	egg yolk	$1\frac{1}{4}$
Lauric isopropanolamide	1	Water	$68\frac{1}{4}$
Fatty alcohol sulphate		Colour essence or	
(paste)	$27\frac{1}{2}$	food dye	A small amount

Method   Mix the egg with a little water to form a paste and then blend this with the ethylene glycol monostearate. Add to the rest of the ingredients and mix thoroughly. To get an egg colour, some yellow-orange colour essence or food dye should be used.

Solid creams

Sodium lauryl sulphate	$12\frac{1}{2}$	Stearic acid	$2\frac{1}{2}$
Sodium hydroxide	$\frac{1}{3}$	Perfume oil	As desired
Diethylene glycol		Water	35
monostearate	1		

Method   Heat the sodium lauryl sulphate with some of the water, stir well, and add the other ingredients, mixing to form a stiff cream shampoo.

Oil-based

Oil-based shampoos give little lather but are good for alleviating dandruff.

(a)		*fluid ounces*	
Sulphonated castor oil	8	Perfume oil	$\frac{1}{4}$
Sulphonated olive oil	8	Water	34

Mineral oil	$1\frac{1}{2}$	Glycerine	$1\frac{1}{2}$
Sulphonated castor oil	$38\frac{1}{2}$	Perfume oil	$\frac{1}{4}$
Oleyl alcohol	$1\frac{1}{2}$	Water	7

Method Mix all the ingredients together so that they are well blended.

Medicated

Various substances can be added to produce medicated shampoos. They include menthol, camphor, thymol, coal tar, pine oil etc. Here is a typical example, using thymol:

Thymol	$\frac{1}{10}$	Water	$49\frac{3}{4}$
Triethanolamine lauryl sulphate	50		

Method Dissolve the thymol in a small amount of alcohol and add this to the other ingredients, blending well.

Note Only similar small quantities should be used if other items, such as coal tar or menthol, are preferred.

Hairdressings and perm lotions

Setting lotions

A simple setting lotion may be prepared by mixing $\frac{1}{2}$ fluid ounce of raw egg white with 2 fluid ounces of warm water. Comb this through your hair and set it. More sophisticated recipes include:

(a)

Gum tragacanth	$\frac{5}{8}$	Alcohol	5
Glycerine	$2\frac{1}{2}$	Water	$41\frac{1}{2}$

(b)

Gum karaya	$\frac{3}{4}$	Glycerine	$2\frac{1}{2}$
Alcohol	5	Water	41
Borax	$\frac{3}{4}$		

(c)

Irish moss	1	Water	49

Perfume oil and colouring in small amounts to suit individual taste may be added.

Method   Mix all the ingredients well together.

(d) Powder

Gum acacia	$23\frac{1}{2}$	Sodium carbonate	4
Gum karaya	15	Perfume oil	$\frac{1}{8}$
Borax	$7\frac{1}{2}$		

Method   Crush the ingredients to a fine powder and mix them well together, adding the perfume oil drop by drop.

When using the mixture, dissolve one ounce of the powder in three pints of hot water. Let it cool a little before use.

Permanent waving

Solutions for permanent waving are alkaline. Usually in professional practice the hair is wound on rollers in slight tension and sachets or absorbent strips dipped in the waving solutions wound around the hair. The hair is then steamed for about ten minutes, rinsed and neutralized and shortly afterwards unwound. A further application of neutralizer follows. Then the final rinse is given and the hair is set. Great care must be taken.

Waving solutions

(a)

Sodium carbonate	2	Ammonium hydroxide	10
Potassium sulphite	1	Water	37

(b)

Borax	2	Ammonium hydroxide	7
Potassium sulphite	1	Water	40

Method Dissolve the ingredients in the heated water and stir well. Then use as described in the first paragraph above.

Neutralizing solution

Hydrogen peroxide	4	Water	40

Method Mix the ingredients together. This quantity can be made greater or smaller, according to need, but care must be taken to keep the relative proportions of the ingredients constant.

Cold waving

This is simpler to use than the above method. Home perms need a reducing solution, as given below, and a neutralizer. After shampooing, the hair is moistened with the reducing solution, wound on to rollers, and left for up to forty minutes.

The rinsing, neutralizing and setting is then carried out exactly as described in the first paragraph above.

Reducing solution

Thioglycollic acid	$2\frac{1}{3}$	Water	$30\frac{7}{8}$
Ammonium hydroxide	$\frac{3}{4}$		

Method Mix the ingredients well together.

Hair lacquers

The oldest material used for hair lacquer is shellac, the resin of a scale insect which is deposited on the twigs of trees growing in tropical southern Asia.

(a)

Shellac	20	Alcohol	$95\frac{1}{2}$
Castor oil	1	Perfume oil	$\frac{1}{4}$
Diethyl phthalate	1		

(b)

Shellac	5	Water	64
Triethanolamine	1	Perfume oil	$\frac{1}{2}$
Alcohol	30		

Method Warm the shellac and dissolve it in a little of the alcohol. Mix this solution well with the other ingredients. Apply by spraying.

Note An aerosol spray is the best form of applicator, but home users can make do with a bottle, squeeze-bulb and tube – these are sold as scent sprays.

Brilliantines and creams for men

Traditional men's hair oils and creams are normally more greasy than those used by women. Nowadays the women's type is often preferred by men.

Liquid brilliantines

(a)

Deodorized kerosene or paraffin	20	Light mineral oil	30

(b)

Light mineral oil	$37\frac{1}{2}$	Lanolin	$\frac{1}{2}$
Isopropyl myristate	12		

Method Mix well, adding a small amount of perfume oil and colouring, if desired.

Alcoholic brilliantines

Alcoholic brilliantines are made by mixing castor oil with alcohol, for instance 20 fluid ounces of castor oil well blended with 80 fluid ounces of industrial alcohol and about $\frac{1}{2}$ fluid ounce of a perfume oil such as rose geranium or lavender.

Solid brilliantines

(a)

Petroleum jelly	$37\frac{1}{2}$	Light mineral oil	$7\frac{1}{2}$
Paraffin wax	$2\frac{1}{2}$	Perfume oil	$\frac{1}{4}$
Microcrystalline wax	$2\frac{1}{2}$	Colour	As desired

(b)

Carnauba wax	$2\frac{1}{2}$	Mineral oil	10
Petroleum jelly	35	Perfume oil	$\frac{1}{4}$
Paraffin wax	$2\frac{1}{2}$	Colour	As desired

(c) Transparent brilliantine

Aluminium stearate	$2\frac{1}{8}$	Castor oil (optional)	5
Light paraffin oil	$47\frac{1}{2}$	Perfume oil	As desired

Method　Heat all the ingredients, stir well until thoroughly blended and then cool slowly.

Note　Two-solution brilliantines consist of equal parts of mineral oil and alcohol with perfume oil and colouring. The layers remain separate and the container holding them must be well shaken before use.

Hair creams

(a)

White mineral oil	$22\frac{1}{2}$	Perfume oil	$\frac{1}{8}$
Triethanolamine	$\frac{3}{4}$	Water	25
Stearic acid	$1\frac{3}{4}$		

(b)

Mineral oil	$16\frac{1}{2}$	Borax	$\frac{1}{8}$
Beeswax	$1\frac{1}{2}$	Triethanolamine	$\frac{7}{8}$
Stearic acid	$\frac{1}{4}$	Water	30
Cetyl alcohol	$\frac{5}{8}$	Perfume oil	$\frac{1}{4}$

Beeswax	$\frac{3}{4}$	Calcium hydroxide	$\frac{1}{5}$
Liquid paraffin	20	Magnesium sulphate	$\frac{1}{4}$
Oleic acid	$\frac{1}{2}$	Perfume oil	$\frac{1}{4}$

(d)

Petroleum jelly	$3\frac{3}{4}$	Borax	$\frac{1}{4}$
Mineral oil	$18\frac{3}{4}$	Sorbitan sesquioleate	$1\frac{1}{2}$
Lanolin	$1\frac{1}{2}$	Water	$23\frac{1}{2}$
Beeswax	1	Perfume oil	$\frac{1}{4}$

(e)

Mineral oil	18	Lime water	19
Petroleum jelly	$1\frac{1}{2}$	Sorbitan sesquioleate	$\frac{1}{3}$
Beeswax	1	Perfume oil	$\frac{1}{4}$
Stearic acid	$\frac{1}{5}$		

(f)

Beeswax	1	Wool wax alcohol	$\frac{1}{3}$
Mineral oil	15	Lime water	$29\frac{1}{2}$
Petroleum jelly	4	Perfume oil	$\frac{1}{4}$
Stearic acid	$\frac{1}{10}$		

Method Heat the oils and waxes, mixing well. Add the water and other ingredients to form a well-blended cream, stirring continuously. Add the perfume oil when nearly cool.

Cream for women's hair

(a)

Mineral oil	$12\frac{1}{2}$	Polyethylene glycol	
Deodorized kerosene		200 stearate	$4\frac{1}{2}$
(paraffin)	$12\frac{1}{2}$		

Polyethylene glycol oleate	$1\frac{1}{2}$	Water	19
		Perfume oil	$\frac{1}{4}$

(b)

Mineral oil	$1\frac{3}{4}$	Cetavlon or cetrimide	$1\frac{1}{2}$
Cetostearyl alcohol	$7\frac{1}{2}$	Water	$39\frac{1}{4}$
Lanolin	$\frac{3}{4}$	Perfume oil	$\frac{1}{4}$

Method Prepare as the other hair creams already mentioned.

Hair fixatives or non-oily dressing

Gum tragacanth	$\frac{1}{2}$	Glycerine	$\frac{1}{2}$
Alcohol	3	Water	45
Castor oil	1	Perfume oil	$\frac{1}{4}$

Method Disperse the gum tragacanth in the alcohol and add the other ingredients, heating as necessary and stirring well. The perfume oil should be added before the mixture is cool.

Bay rum

This originally contained rum, but cheaper forms are made from methylated spirits and water.

Oil of bay	1	Water	14
Rum or industrial alcohol	24	Glycerine (optional)	$\frac{3}{4}$

Method Mix all the ingredients together.

Hair conditioner

| Avocado | ½ fruit | Eggs | 2 |
| *or* avocado oil | ⅛ fluid ounce | | |

Method Mix well together, beating to a froth. Apply well to hair, massaging it in. Leave for a quarter of an hour, then rinse after working it to a lather on the hair with some warm water. Rinse finally with lots of water.

Colorants and bleaches

The materials from which these products are made should have no toxic effects nor have any irritating action on the hair or skin. Vegetable dyes are very safe for general use. Commercial hair dyes are of vegetable, metallic or synthetic origin.

Vegetable hair dyes

Henna This is made from powdered leaves of the plants *Lawsonia alba*, *Lawsonia spinosa* and *Lawsonia inermis*. When mixed with hot water to a paste and applied to the hair for up to an hour, henna produces a reddish-auburn colour.

Henna Reng Mixtures of powdered indigo leaves, from the *Indigofera* plant family, and henna leaves, yielding blueish-black shades. These are popular in the Far East.

Lysimachia This is the plant *Lythrum salicaria*, the perennial purple willow herb or loosestrife. The dried leaves and shoots are used to give a blonde tint to the hair. Apply as for henna.

Corisson Produced by the plant *Lythrum hypericon* (sometimes known as *Hypericon perforatum*), the perforated

St John's Wort, which is quite common especially in lime soils. It colours the hair black.

Ophrys The eyebrow plant, called botanically *Ophrys ovata* or *bifolia*. It produces a black dye.

Jacob's Ladder Called botanically *Polemonium caeruleum*, this plant, when boiled in oil, produces a good black dye.

Camomile Roman camomile is known botanically as *Anthemis nobilis* and German camomile as *Matricaria chamomillae*. After drying and grinding up the flower heads, make them into a paste with hot water and an equal quantity of powdered kaolin. Mix these ingredients to form a thin cream. Apply to the hair and follow by a very quick rinse (not a shampoo). To lighten your natural hair colour, leave on for a quarter of an hour; to obtain a warm blonde tint allow up to one hour. Camomile is also used to brighten and enliven hair.

Unhappily, vegetable hair dyes have been generally replaced today in commercial preparations by metallic or synthetic materials, which are more economic.

Metallic hair dyes

These hair dyes are made from compounds of lead, silver, copper, iron, nickel and bismuth. They may make hair brittle and give it a dull appearance. Metallic dyes normally work slowly and tinting is progressive over weeks or even months.

For grey hair

(a)

Lead acetate	1	Alcohol	20
Sodium thiosulphate	3	Water	160
Glycerine	16	Perfume	As desired

87

(b)

Precipitated sulphur	10	Water	157
Lead acetate	3	Perfume	As desired
Glycerine	30		

Mixture Mix well and keep in dark or amber coloured bottles. Use the mixture on the hair only and not on the scalp.

Silver dyes These are solution types, which colour the hair various shades from ash blonde to brown and black, according to the amount of silver present in the formula. Before using the silver dye, cold cream or vaseline must be applied to the forehead, ears and neck, to stop the skin being stained black from any dye accidentally falling on it.

Darker shades

Silver nitrate	4	Ammonium	
Copper sulphate	$\frac{1}{5}$	hydroxide	As required
Water	110		

Method Mix the ingredients, first crushing any lumps to a fine powder. The residues or precipitate in the solution are then redissolved by slowly adding small amounts of the ammonium hydroxide, to produce a lotion.

Lighter shades *(less silver)*

Silver nitrate	$2\frac{1}{2}$	Ammonium	
Nickel sulphate	$\frac{1}{10}$	hydroxide	As required
Water	110		

Method Prepare as above. Use distilled water or rainwater, if uncontaminated.

88

Brown tint

Pyrogallic acid	10	Water	70
Ammonia solution	5	Perfume	As desired
Alcohol	25		

Method Mix and apply. Bottled ammonia solution is available in chemists' shops.

Chestnut shade

Pyrogallic acid	5	Alcohol	29
Glacial acetic acid	1	Water	70

Method Mix and apply.

Ash-blonde shade

Pyrogallic acid	1	Sodium sulphite	2
Cobalt nitrate	$\frac{1}{2}$	Water	$46\frac{1}{2}$

Method Mix and apply.

Synthetic hair dyes

Temporary, semi-permanent and permanent dyes are used commercially. Water rinses or temporary colorants usually contain dyestuff and tartaric or citric acid.

Rinses

(a)

Colour dyestuff	1	Tartaric acid	19

Method Mix in warm water to use.

(b)

Dyestuff	3	Citric acid	20
Alcohol	5	Water	22

Lighteners and bleaches

There are bleaching pastes and powders as well as liquids and creams for lightening hair.

Only bleach any lot of hair once. Repeated bleaching of the same strands produces a straw-like appearance and damages the hair texture badly. Take care to bleach only new growths of hair on an already bleached head, and not the previously treated growth.

Simple bleach

After shampooing well and drying the hair, take 2 fluid ounces of hydrogen peroxide and add to this $\frac{1}{24}$ fluid ounce (40 drops or $\frac{3}{4}$ of a teaspoonful) of ammonium hydroxide, mixing well. Divide the hair into small portions and apply the mixture to the full length of it, portion by portion. Rinse with lots of cool water. Hydrogen peroxide in 6 per cent solution is available in chemists' shops.

For a platinum blonde effect, rinse the hair after bleaching with a blue rinse containing methylene blue or other certified blue colour. The proportions are one part of the methylene blue to 100,000 of water.

Shampoo bleach

To 8 fluid ounces of a good shampoo add 4 fluid ounces of hydrogen peroxide and $\frac{1}{12}$ of a fluid ounce of ammonium hydroxide. Wash your hair in this, leave on for five minutes and rinse. Repeat as necessary.

Bleach powder

Ammonium bicarbonate	2	Magnesium carbonate	5
Ammonium bisulphate	1	Calcium carbonate	2

Method Mix with 10 fluid ounces of hydrogen peroxide to make the bleach.

Liquid bleach

Alcohol	$20\frac{1}{3}$	Triethanolamine	$6\frac{1}{4}$
Oleic acid	$8\frac{1}{4}$	Sodium lauryl ether	
Ammonium hydroxide	$10\frac{1}{4}$	sulphate	$4\frac{3}{4}$

Method Mix well together to form a cream. To use, take a quantity and add to it four times as much by weight of hydrogen peroxide, to give a lotion.

Miscellaneous

To make dull white hair less conspicuous, use sage tea. Infuse *dried sage leaves* in boiling water and apply the liquid to the hair.

Walnut leaves and the *green nutshells* produce a brown hair colorant. Infuse in boiling water and apply to the hair.

Oak nut galls or *oakapples* may be used in a similar way. *Fustic* is produced from the wood of the tree *Chlorophora tinctoria,* which is related to the mulberry. It gives yellow to brown shades.

Various other plants yield dyes of different colours: *Rhubarb,* when combined with henna, black tea and camomile will give a good blonde shade.

Rastik

Mix together 2 pounds of oak nut galls, $\frac{1}{2}$ ounce of copper filings and 1 ounce of iron filings and place them in a roasting tin with a little vegetable cooking oil. Cook until the nut galls are well done. Cool and grind to a fine powder. Add enough water to make a paste and apply this to the hair for several hours. It should produce a beautiful, permanent black.

Hair straighteners

Here is a formula for permanent straightening of kinky hair:

Stearic acid	3	Thioglycollic acid	$61\frac{3}{5}$
Glyceryl monostearate	15	Ammonium hydroxide	20
Ceresine	$1\frac{1}{2}$	Perfume oil	As desired
Paraffin	1	Water	$51\frac{7}{8}$
Sodium lauryl sulphate	1		

Method Heat the glyceryl monostearate, the stearic acid, the paraffin, the ceresine and the sodium lauryl sulphate with just under half of the water, stirring constantly. At the same time, put the thioglycollic acid in the rest of the water and add this solution slowly to the ammonium hydroxide. This generates considerable heat, so keep the pot in a bowl of iced water. Now very slowly pour the mixture of water, thioglycollic acid and ammonium hydroxide into the first mixture of the other ingredients. Mix well, do not let the temperature rise over 122°F (50°C), add the perfume oil and cool. Pack in closed jars.

Note Hair straightener should not be used if you have cuts or abrasions on your head, or if your hair is in poor condition. Wash your hair before the straightener is applied.

The straightener should not be allowed to drop on the skin, and some petroleum jelly should be smeared on the forehead and the ears, or on any other exposed areas, to protect them.

When employing this recipe, a neutralizer must be poured over the hair for several minutes after the straightener has completed its work. Finally, rinse well with plain cool water.

Neutralizer

Sodium bromate	14	Sorbitan trioleate	2
Propylene glycol	2	Sodium cetyl sulphate	3
Lanolin	2	Water	76
Sorbitan monopalmitate	1	Perfume oil	As desired

Method Dissolve the sodium bromate in the water and the propylene glycol, using heat. Then mix the other ingredients and add them. Stir well, cool, add perfume oil and pack.

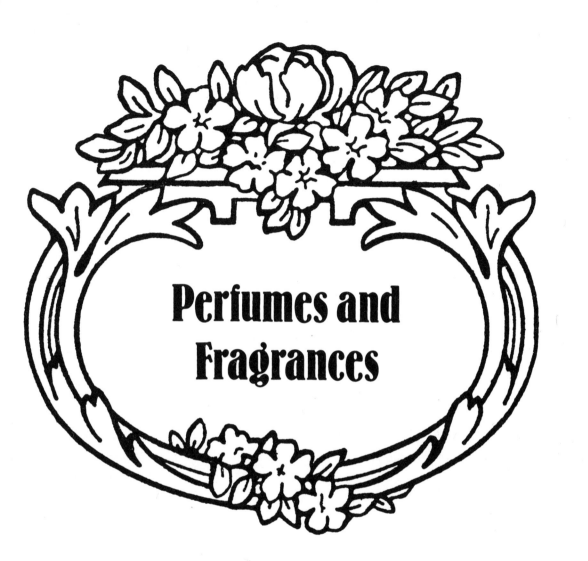

Perfumes and Fragrances

The basic ingredients

Perfumes are mixtures or blends of various raw materials, in particular essential, aromatic, ethereal or perfume oils, flower oils, gums and resins, animal secretions, and chemical substances mainly derived from plants or synthetic organic products.

Simple mixtures contain about six constituents, but in commercially made scents and perfumes there are often twenty to thirty, and at times well over one hundred ingredients.

Important essential oils

Name	Odour
Citronella	Lemon-like
Lemon grass	Lemon-like
Lavender	Lavender
Lavadin }	{ Lavender
Spike lavender }	or lavender-like
Rosemary	Herby and camphor-like
Orange	Orange
Lemon	Lemon
Lime	Sharp, lemonlike
Bergamot	Orange-like
Petitgrain	Orange-like
Bois de Rose	Fresh, woody rose
Sandalwood	Sandalwood, woody
Cedarwood	Woody
Vetivert	Heavy, sweet, vegetable-like
Patchouli	Spicy, camphor-like

Geranium	Rose or mint-like
Clove	Spicy, clove
Ylang-ylang	Flowery
Otto of rose	Rose petal
Oakmoss (resinoid)	Mossy, earthy
Carnation	Flowery
Cassie (absolute and concrete)	Orange-violet-cumin
Gardenia (absolute and concrete)	Tuberose-jasmin-orange
Jasmine (absolute and concrete)	Jasmine
Lilac (absolute)	Indigo-jasmin-hawthorn or may blossom
Lily (absolute and concrete)	Lily, honey-like
Narcissus (absolute and concrete)	Flowery
Neroli	Orange-like
Sweet pea	Orange-rose-hyacinth
Tuberose (absolute)	Flowery, assorted
Violet (absolute and concrete)	Violet

Many others are listed on page 159.

Animal products

Name	Origin
Ambergris	Sperm whale
Musk	Gland of musk deer
Civet	Secretion from civet cat
Castoreum	Gland of beaver

Synthetics Simulated odours, often cheaper than natural products and not so subject to market price changes or lack of consistency in supply.

Alcohols Blending agents.

Making and building up a perfume

Simple perfumes can be made up by following basic formulae, but to build up 'fantasy' perfumes requires imagination. Perfumery is therefore called an art and its professional practitioners are highly regarded in their own circles. This, of course, means that home makers of scents can exercise their individual talents and construct their own formulae, experimenting as they go. It can be a fascinating and instructive hobby. Here are some simple recipes for perfumes:

Perfumes

Esterhazy

Orange flower	1	Neroli	1
Rose	1	Sandalwood	$\frac{1}{16}$
Vetivert	1	Clove	$\frac{1}{16}$
Vanilla	1	Ambergris	$\frac{1}{2}$
Orris	1	Alcohol	1 pint or
Tonka	1		as desired

Eau de Cologne

Neroli	1	Ciste	$1\frac{1}{5}$
Rosemary	$\frac{1}{2}$	Bergamot	$\frac{1}{2}$
Orange	$1\frac{1}{5}$	Alcohol	Up to 1 gallon

Millefleurs

Lemon	1	Lavender	$\frac{3}{4}$

Clove	$\frac{3}{4}$	Ambergris	Enough to cover the head of a pin
Verbena	$\frac{1}{20}$		
Pimento	$\frac{1}{20}$	Musk	Enough to cover the head of a pin
Neroli	$\frac{1}{20}$		
Styrax	$\frac{1}{12}$	Alcohol	Up to 2–3 pints

Bouquet d'Amour

Jasmine	2	Musk	1
Rose	2	Ambergris	1
Violet	2	Alcohol	Up to $\frac{1}{2}$ pint
Cassie	2		

Fleur

Jonquil	$7\frac{1}{2}$	Ylang-ylang	1
Jasmine	1	Bitter almond	$2\frac{1}{2}$
Tuberose	2	Wintergreen	$\frac{1}{2}$
Cassie	1	Angelica	3 drops
Orange	1	Styrax	$\frac{5}{8}$
Bergamot	$\frac{1}{10}$	Musk	$\frac{1}{8}$
Lemon	$\frac{1}{20}$	Alcohol	Up to $\frac{1}{2}$ pint
Vanilla	$\frac{1}{2}$		

Bouquet des Fleurs

Bergamot	8	Rose	5
Lemon	4	Benzoin	$2\frac{1}{3}$
Orange	4	Alcohol	As required for dilution
Violet	5		
Tuberose	5		

Rose of the Fields

Bergamot	4	Mace	4
Jasmine	5	Civet	$\frac{1}{4}$
Rose	6	Alcohol	As required
Tuberose	$3\frac{1}{2}$		

Garden of Flowers

Cassie	5	Rose	5
Jonquil	10	Citronella	$\frac{1}{8}$
Coumarin	$\frac{1}{2}$	Lemon grass	$\frac{1}{2}$
Paracresyl		Ambergris	1
phenylacetate	$\frac{1}{4}$	Civet	$\frac{3}{4}$
Orris	$\frac{1}{2}$	Alcohol	As required

Musk

Musk ambrette	4	Sandalwood	2
Musk ketone	4	Benzyl benzoate	8
Ionone beta	1	Alcohol	As required
Vetivert	1		

Polyanthus

Rose	6	Lemon	4
Jasmine	3	Musk	$1\frac{1}{2}$
Violet	$1\frac{1}{2}$	Alcohol	As required

Rondeletia

Bergamot	6	Lavender	$12\frac{1}{2}$
Basil	$\frac{1}{2}$	Clove	$2\frac{1}{2}$

Rose	1	Jasmine	$\frac{1}{2}$
Sandalwood	15	Tuberose	$\frac{1}{2}$
Geranium	2	Vanillin	1
Cinnamon leaf	2	Musk ketone	$1\frac{1}{2}$
Ambrette	$\frac{1}{2}$	Ambergris	$3\frac{1}{2}$
Orris	1	Alcohol	As required

Fresh Breeze

Orange	5	Vanillin	$1\frac{1}{4}$
Jasmine	2	Rose	$2\frac{1}{2}$
Cassie	$\frac{1}{2}$	Benzoin	$8\frac{1}{8}$
Sandalwood	5	Alcohol	As required

A la Mode

Nutmeg	$\frac{3}{4}$	Tuberose	$5\frac{1}{2}$
Cassie	3	Benzaldehyde	$\frac{1}{4}$
Jasmine	$8\frac{1}{4}$	Civet	$\frac{1}{2}$
Orange	$5\frac{1}{2}$	Alcohol	As required

Essence Bouquet

Petitgrain	4	Thyme	$\frac{1}{2}$
Sweet orange	4	Palmarosa	$\frac{1}{3}$
Rose	$3\frac{3}{4}$	Clove	$\frac{1}{4}$
Jasmine	$3\frac{1}{4}$	Cassia	$\frac{1}{4}$
Lavender	3	Musk	$\frac{1}{4}$
Lemon	2	Alcohol	As required
Neroli	2		

Eau de Berlin

Aniseed	$\frac{1}{2}$	Neroli	$\frac{2}{3}$
Bergamot	12	Sandalwood	$\frac{1}{3}$
Cardamon	$\frac{1}{4}$	Thyme	$\frac{1}{4}$
Coriander	$\frac{1}{5}$	Ethyl phthalate	10
Geranium	$\frac{1}{3}$	Rhodinol	$\frac{1}{2}$
Lemon	$\frac{1}{3}$	Alcohol	As required
Melissa (balm)	$\frac{1}{4}$		

Hovenia

Lemon	$4\frac{1}{8}$	Iso-eugenol	$6\frac{3}{4}$
Petitgrain	$4\frac{1}{4}$	Alcohol	As required
Rose	$4\frac{1}{4}$		

Japanese Bouquet

Cedarwood	4	Vetivert	2
Patchouli	4	Rose	7
Sandalwood	4	Alcohol	As required
Verbena	4		

Leap year

Jasmine	6	Verbena	$\frac{3}{4}$
Patchouli	$\frac{1}{2}$	Vetivert	3
Sandalwood	3	Rose	3
Tuberose	4	Alcohol	As required

Bouquet à la Marechale

Neroli	5	Rose	10
Orange	10	Clove	2
Coumarin	4	Sandalwood	2
Vanillin	4	Musk	2
Orris	4	Ambergris	2
Vetivert	5	Alcohol	As desired

Tulip

Cassie	2	Orris	13
Jasmine	13	Neroli	$1\frac{1}{2}$
Rose	$6\frac{3}{4}$	Benzaldehyde	$\frac{3}{4}$
Tuberose	13	Alcohol	As desired

Chypre

Ambrette	5	Geraniol	$\frac{1}{30}$
Tonka	$12\frac{1}{2}$	Musk	15
Vanillin	$7\frac{1}{2}$	Alcohol	As required
Orris	$7\frac{1}{2}$		

Purple Lilac

Vanillin	5	Lemon	5 drops
Orris	10	Bergamot	5 drops
Orange	20	Bitter almond	1 drop
Jasmine	20	Styrax	$\frac{1}{8}$
Tuberose	10	Alcohol	As required
Cassie	5		

Santolina

Lavender	4	Vetivert	$\frac{5}{8}$
Bergamot	1	Cassie	$\frac{5}{8}$
Ylang-ylang	$\frac{3}{4}$	Rose	$1\frac{1}{2}$
Clary sage	$\frac{1}{4}$	Benzoin	$1\frac{1}{4}$
Oakmoss	$\frac{1}{10}$	Alcohol	As required
Ambrette	$\frac{1}{2}$		

Bouquet des Alpes

Lavender	4	Rosemary	$\frac{1}{4}$
Bergamot	1	Jasmine	$\frac{1}{2}$
Geraniol	1	Ethyl phthalate	$\frac{7}{8}$
Ambrette	$\frac{1}{20}$	Benzoin	2
Ylang-ylang	$\frac{1}{4}$	Alcohol	As required
Clary sage	$\frac{1}{20}$		

Violet

Violet	14	Musk	$\frac{1}{2}$
Cassie	$\frac{1}{2}$	Civet	$\frac{1}{10}$
Rose	$\frac{1}{10}$	Ambergris	$\frac{1}{4}$
Sandalwood	$\frac{1}{5}$	Alcohol	As required

Acacia

Bergamot	5	Sandalwood	1
Bitter almond	1	Methyl cinnamate	2
Ylang-ylang	4	Iso-eugenol	1
Orange	2	Musk	3
Jasmine	2	Alcohol	As required
Rose	$1\frac{1}{4}$		

Note The amounts of alcohol added to formulae can be adjusted to suit individual taste and needs.

Toilet waters

Honey water

(a)

Honey	10	Gum benzoin	$\frac{1}{2}$
Corianders	10	Alcohol	As required
Cloves	$\frac{3}{4}$		(usually $\frac{1}{2}$ pint)
Nutmegs	$\frac{1}{2}$	Orange oil	$\frac{1}{2}$
Vanilla essence	$\frac{1}{2}$	Rose oil	$\frac{1}{2}$
Lemon essence	1	Musk	$\frac{1}{10}$
Styrax	$\frac{1}{2}$	Ambergris	$\frac{1}{10}$

Method Grind up the materials, add the essences and dissolve in the alcohol. Leave for a few weeks in a closed jar. Then add the orange oil, rose oil, musk and ambergris, after breaking up the last two into powder. Mix well and heat for three days at a slow simmer, in a pan with a lid. Then cool, filter and bottle.

(b)

Honey	$2\frac{1}{2}$	Sandalwood oil	$1\frac{3}{4}$
Bergamot oil	4	Musk	1
Lavender oil	$\frac{1}{2}$	Benzoin	$2\frac{1}{2}$
Clove oil	$\frac{1}{2}$	Rosewater	50
Nutmeg oil	$\frac{1}{4}$	Orange flower water	50
Coriander oil	$\frac{1}{2}$	Alcohol	400

Method Mix together and leave for six months in a closed jar. Filter before use.

Hungary water

Rosemary oil	1	Peppermint oil	$\frac{1}{4}$
Verbena oil	$3\frac{1}{2}$	Rose water	50
Orange oil	$\frac{3}{4}$	Orange flower water	50
Lime oil	$\frac{1}{2}$	Alcohol	400

Method Prepare by mixing the ingredients and keep for six months. Filter before use.

Eau de Cologne

There are many formulae for Eau de Cologne. Here are a few simple ones.

(a)

Bergamot oil	4	Neroli oil	$1\frac{1}{4}$
Lemon oil	3	Rosemary oil	$\frac{1}{4}$
Sweet orange oil	$2\frac{1}{2}$	Benzoin	$2\frac{1}{2}$
Lavender oil	$\frac{1}{2}$	Alcohol	250
Orris	5		

(b)

Neroli oil	$2\frac{1}{2}$	Lavender oil	$\frac{1}{4}$
Bergamot oil	6	Orange flower water	25
Lemon oil	3	Ambergris	$2\frac{1}{2}$
Rosemary oil	$\frac{1}{2}$	Alcohol	475
Origanum oil	$\frac{1}{4}$		

(c) Amber Cologne

Lemon oil	$2\frac{1}{2}$	Bois de Rose oil	$2\frac{1}{2}$
Bergamot oil	5	Rosemary oil	$\frac{1}{2}$
Mandarin oil	$2\frac{1}{2}$	Coumarin	$1\frac{1}{2}$

Vanillin	1	Neroli oil	$1\frac{3}{4}$
Benzoin resin	$2\frac{1}{2}$	Ambergris	$12\frac{1}{2}$
Ethyl cinnamate	$\frac{3}{4}$	Benzoin	$2\frac{1}{2}$
Clary sage oil	$\frac{1}{2}$	Alcohol	500

(d)

Bergamot oil	20	Rosemary oil	$2\frac{1}{2}$
Lemon oil	2	Orange flower water	30
Neroli oil	$3\frac{1}{2}$	Alcohol	600
Origanum oil	1		

Method   Mix the ingredients and place in a closed container and mature for six months. This ensures the correct strength and odour in the finished product. After maturation, filter and bottle.

Lavender water

(a)

Lavender oil	10	Orris	$2\frac{1}{2}$
Bergamot oil	5	Alcohol	500
Musk	$2\frac{1}{2}$		

Method   Mix, place in a closed container and mature for six months. Then filter and bottle.

(b) Quicker-maturing

Lavender oil	30	Oakmoss	$\frac{1}{8}$
Bergamot oil	$12\frac{1}{2}$	Patchouli oil	$\frac{1}{8}$
Neroli oil	1	Coumarin	$\frac{1}{2}$
Rose oil	$\frac{1}{2}$	Musk	$\frac{1}{4}$
Orris	1	Civet	$\frac{1}{4}$
Vanilla essence	$2\frac{1}{2}$	Alcohol	500

Method Dissolve the materials in the alcohol and leave in a closed container for a month. Then filter and bottle.

(c) Amber lavender

Lavender oil	10	Musk ambrette	$\frac{1}{2}$
Bergamot oil	5	Castoreum	$2\frac{1}{2}$
Lemon oil	1	Ambergris	$12\frac{1}{2}$
Clary sage oil	$1\frac{1}{2}$	Alcohol	500

Method Prepare as for *(a)* above.

Florida water

Neroli oil	$2\frac{1}{2}$	Cinnamon oil	$\frac{1}{2}$
Lavender oil	$3\frac{1}{2}$	Rose otto	$2\frac{1}{2}$
Bergamot oil	15	Ambergris	1
Lime oil	1	Orange flower water	50
Clove oil	1	Alcohol	450
Cassia oil	$\frac{1}{2}$		

Method Mix well together and mature for six months in a closed container. Then filter and bottle.

Eau de Cananga

Cananga oil	$2\frac{1}{2}$	Musk	1
Bergamot oil	2	Benzaldehyde	$\frac{1}{20}$
Lemon oil	$\frac{1}{2}$	Alcohol	As required

Eau de Portugal

Sweet orange oil	10	Rose geranium oil	$\frac{1}{2}$
Bergamot oil	3	Benzoin	1
Lemon oil	$1\frac{1}{2}$	Alcohol	As required

Method Prepare as for the other toilet waters.

Rosewater

The roses which yield perfume for scents are the Rose de Mai or cabbage rose, *Rosa centifolia;* the Damascene rose, *Rosa damascena,* as well as Rose de l'Hay, a crossbred; the white rose, *Rosa alba,* which may also be pale pink; and the Provence rose, *Rosa gallica,* sometimes called the damask rose.

To prepare rosewater at home, quantities of petals should be macerated (mashed and warmed in a little sesame oil to extract the scent). After straining, this oil can be mixed with distilled water to individual taste.

Orange water

Several varieties of oranges are used for oil production and it is during the distillation process that commercial orange flower water is obtained as a by-product. Orange flower absolute can be mixed with water to make orange flower water.

Solid perfumes

Fragrance vehicles, such as solid perfumes or sticks and sachets, as well as potpourris, are not difficult to prepare.

Potpourri

(a)

Lavender flowers	10	Mace	1
Red or other scented		Calamus root	5
rose petals	40	Benzoin, Siam	3
Coarse sandalwood	20	Coriander seeds	2
Coarse orris rhizome	5	Rose oil	1
Patchouli leaves	3	Neroli oil	1
Vetivert leaves	1	Jasmine oil absolute	1
Tonka beans	1	Ambergris	1
Cloves	2	Heliotropin	1
Cinnamon bark	1	*or* Heliotrope leaves	10
Allspice	1		

Method   Mix well together and store in a closed container.

(b)

Fresh rose petals	35	Salt	2

Method   Mix and leave for five days, then add the following ingredients and store in a closed container:

Powdered orris root	1	Petals of any sweet scented	
Allspice	1	flowers available, such as	
Cloves	1	heliotrope or mignonette	
Rosemary	$\frac{1}{2}$	etc.	5
Bay leaves	$\frac{1}{4}$	Brandy	$1\frac{1}{2}$
Verbena oil	$\frac{1}{4}$		

(c)

Dried rose petals	35	Scented geranium	
Bay leaves	$\frac{1}{4}$	blossoms	4
Clover heads	5	Delphinium petals	2

Mock orange blossom flowers	2	Orange peel, chopped up	2
Lavender leaves or heads	4	Lemon peel, chopped up	2
Laurel leaves	2	Mint leaves	$\frac{1}{2}$
Red wallflowers or gillyflowers	3		

Method Mix well and allow to dry slowly. Then add the following ingredients and mix well. Store to mature in a closed jar.

Powdered cinnamon	1	Mace	1
Ground-up cloves	1	Salt	1
Allspice	1	Sea salt or bay salt	1

Olla Podrida is a sort of 'dog's breakfast' of all left-over scented or aromatic materials, with the addition of leaves of herbs such as rosemary, thyme, lavender, flower petals of different kinds, and a little alcohol, well mixed together and matured. It is used for similar purposes as potpourri.

Sachets are made up of scented and aromatic materials, stitched into silk or velvet envelopes.

Solids

White beeswax	2	Ethyl phthalate	4
Japan wax	2	Perfume oils of choice	2

Method Mix together.

The amounts of the waxes and the ethyl phthalate may be varied to give softer or harder perfume sticks or pomades.

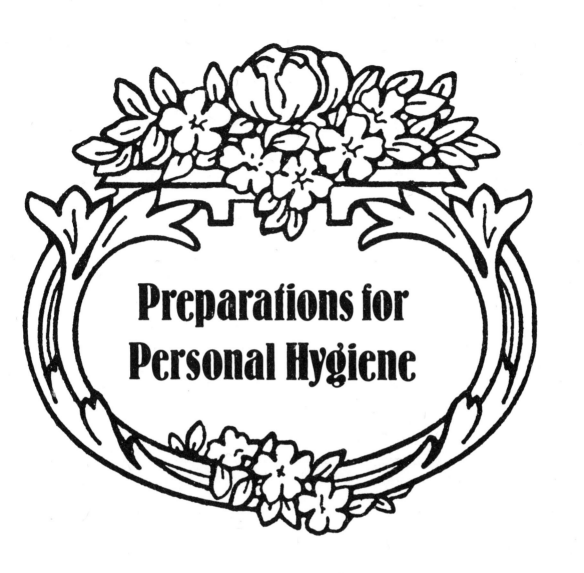

Preparations for
Personal Hygiene

Dentifrices

These are toothpastes and tooth powders for cleaning the teeth. A good dentifrice should assist the toothbrush, make the mouth feel fresh and pleasant, be reasonably cheap, and safe. The prices of many commercial toothpastes and powders today bear little relation to the costs of the ingredients. Preservatives can be used, as with other products.

Toothpastes

(a)

Calcium carbonate	40	Saccharin sodium	$\frac{1}{20}$
Glycerine	30	Sodium lauryl sulphate	$1\frac{1}{5}$
Mineral oil	1	Water	$21\frac{1}{2}$
Propylene glycol	5	Additional flavour	
Gum tragacanth	$1\frac{1}{5}$		As desired

(b)

Dicalcium phosphate	60	Gum tragacanth	1
Glycerine	$7\frac{1}{2}$	Water	11
Sodium lauryl sulphate	$2\frac{1}{2}$	Flavour	As desired
Propylene glycol	$17\frac{1}{2}$		

(c)

Chalk	$28\frac{1}{2}$	Gum tragacanth	$\frac{3}{4}$
Glycerine	$10\frac{1}{2}$	Water	$9\frac{1}{2}$
Sodium lauryl sulphate	$\frac{1}{2}$	Flavour	As desired

Method   Small amounts of different essential oils may be

added to the toothpaste mixtures, for instance peppermint, spearmint, cinnamon, caraway, wintergreen, also menthol, to give special tastes and flavours. Saccharin is a flavour and sweetener. Chlorophyll may reduce breath odour. Fluorine may check tooth decay.

When preparing toothpastes, the gum should be made into a mucilage with the water and glycerine, warming it if necessary, then add the other ingredients, blending and mixing them all well together. Store in closed containers.

Fluoride toothpaste

Fluoride toothpaste generally contains stannous fluoride and calcium pyrophosphate as the polishing agent.

Stannous fluoride	1	Glycerine	75
Calcium pyrophosphate	$97\frac{1}{4}$	Stannous pyrophosphate	$2\frac{1}{4}$

Method Mix the ingredients and add calcium carbonate, flavouring and water to make a good paste.

Tooth powders

(a) For smokers

Precipitated chalk	$9\frac{1}{2}$	Powdered pumice	
Kaolin	$1\frac{1}{2}$	stone	1
Sodium lauryl sulphate	3	Flavour	As desired

(b)

Calcium carbonate	10	Flavour	As desired
Camphor	1		

115

(c)

Calcium carbonate	4	Carbolic acid	$\frac{1}{40}$
Kieselguhr	$5\frac{3}{4}$	Flavour	As desired

(d)

Calcium carbonate	5	Sodium benzoate	$\frac{1}{2}$
Kieselguhr	4	Flavour	As desired
Dental soap powder	$\frac{1}{2}$		

Solid dentifrice

Calcium carbonate	$2\frac{1}{2}$	Glycerine	$\frac{1}{2}$
Dental soap chips		Flavour	As desired
or powder	7		

Cleansers and liquids

(a)

Sodium lauryl sulphate	1	Water	94
Alcohol	$2\frac{1}{2}$	Flavour	As desired

A good flavouring can be made from a mixture of peppermint oil, thymol, anise oil, cinnamon oil and clove oil – a few drops of each – to suit individual taste, and some colour, if desired.

(b)

Boric acid	2	Alcohol	$68\frac{3}{4}$
Phenol	1	Tincture of myrrh	2
Glycerine	$\frac{1}{2}$	Quillaia	10
Rosewater	10	Flavour	As desired

Saccharin sodium may be added to give a sweetening effect.

116

Mouthwashes

(a)

Phenol	$3\frac{3}{4}$	Water	$71\frac{1}{2}$
Sodium hydroxide		Flavour	As desired
(liquid)	$9\frac{3}{4}$	Colouring	
Orange flower water	2	(permanganate	
Glycerine	$12\frac{1}{2}$	of potash)	As desired

Note Sodium hydroxide may be bought as a solution. To use, dilute the mouthwash with five times its volume of warm water.

(b) Glycerine of thymol

Sodium bicarbonate	5	Glycerine	50
Sodium benzoate	4	Alcohol	$12\frac{1}{2}$
Borax	10	Eucalyptus oil	$\frac{3}{4}$
Sodium salicylate	$2\frac{3}{8}$	Pumilionis pine oil	$\frac{1}{4}$
Thymol	$\frac{1}{4}$	Methyl salicylate	$\frac{1}{5}$
Menthol	$\frac{1}{5}$	Water	83

Method Dissolve the powdered materials in the water, then add the glycerine and the other ingredients, mixing well. Filter and store in a stoppered bottle. Colouring should be added to give a reddish tint, also some flavour. To use, dilute with an equal amount of water.

(c)

Eau de Cologne	$32\frac{1}{2}$	Glycerine	6
Borax	2	Flavour	As desired
Tincture of myrrh	2	Water	$7\frac{1}{2}$

Method Mix and store in a closed container.

Denture cleansers

(a)

Sodium percarbonate	4	Sodium carbonate	2
Sodium chloride	4		

(b)

Sodium perborate	4	Trisodium phosphate	3
Sodium chloride	3	Colour	If desired

Note Tablets are made by using a binder, such as sodium silicate; and tartaric acid can be added to give effervescence.

Powdered charcoal mixed with chalk is also a good cleaner for both natural and false teeth.

Antiperspirants and deodorants

Antiperspirants reduce the amount of sweat secreted and may block the openings of the sweat ducts on the skin surface. Deodorants are based on bactericides or antiseptics that either destroy or inhibit the activity of bacteria.

Liquid antiperspirant

Aluminium chlorhydrate	10	Germicide (antiseptic)	$\frac{1}{20}$
Propylene glycol	$2\frac{1}{2}$	Water	32
Alcohol	5	Perfume oil	As desired

Method Mix and blend well.

Absorbent powder

(a)

Boric acid powder	5	Talc	90
Magnesium carbonate	5	Perfume oil	As desired

(b)

Boric acid powder	15	Talc	210
Salicylic acid	25	Perfume oil	As desired
Starch powder	250		

Method   Mix ingredients together well.

Cream

Aluminium chlorhydrate	10	Glycerine	$1\frac{1}{2}$
Glyceryl monostearate	10	Water	26
Spermaceti	$2\frac{1}{2}$	Perfume oil	As desired

Method   Mix well and store in a closed container. The blending is best done by heating.

Stick

Sodium stearate	7	Alcohol	83
Cetyl alcohol	$1\frac{1}{2}$	Water	3
Propylene glycol	5	Perfume oil	$\frac{1}{4}$
Chlorhexidine diacetate	$\frac{1}{2}$		

Method   Heat all the ingredients together, except the perfume oil, until they are well blended. Cool and then add the perfume oil. Pour into moulds to give a stick-like shape.

119

(d) For hot climates

Sodium stearate	10	Benzyl alcohol	5
Urea	$\frac{1}{4}$	Water	24
Propylene glycol	50	Perfume oil	$\frac{1}{3}$
Chlorhexidine diacetate	$\frac{1}{2}$		

Method Mix the chlorhexidine diacetate in the propylene glycol and add the other ingredients, except the sodium stearate and the benzyl alcohol. When well blended, put in these two items. Heating makes the process easier. The perfume oil is added last and the mixture allowed to cool and transferred to moulds to set.

Bath preparations

Bath salts

(a)

Sodium sesquicarbonate	7	Lemon oil	$\frac{1}{16}$
Verbena oil	$\frac{1}{8}$		

Method Sprinkle the oils over the salt and keep in a closed jar.

(b)

Sodium carbonate	10	Perfume oils	As desired

(c)

Sodium carbonate monohydrate	8	Sodium phosphate	2
		Perfume oils	As desired

(d)

Sodium perborate	$\frac{1}{2}$	Borax	1
Sodium sesquicarbonate	$8\frac{1}{2}$	Perfume oils	As desired

(e)

Sodium sesquicarbonate	9	Perfume oils	As desired
Borax	1		

(f)

ounces

Sodium phosphate	5	Perfume oils	As desired
Sodium chloride	5		

Method   Mix as for *(a)*. Colour dyes can be added to tint the salts.

Oxygenated salts

Sodium chloride	3	Sodium carbonate	
Sodium perborate	10	monohydrate	117
Borax	20	Perfume and colour	
Sodium bicarbonate	50		As desired

Therapeutic salts

(a)

Potassium iodide	$\frac{1}{2}$	Sodium sulphate	45
Potassium bromide	$\frac{3}{4}$	Sodium chloride	125
Potassium chloride	$4\frac{3}{4}$	Perfume oil	If desired
Magnesium sulphate	75		

121

(b)

Magnesium sulphate	6	Sodium chloride	$2\frac{1}{2}$
Sodium sulphate	$1\frac{1}{2}$	Perfume oil	If desired

(c)

Magnesium chloride	1	Magnesium sulphate	109
Sodium thiosulphate	90	Perfume oil	If desired

Magnesium sulphate in the bath water is said to be helpful to rheumatism sufferers and to alleviate sprains and bruises.

Bath powders and cubes

(a)

Sodium sesquicarbonate	8	Borax (powdered)	2

(b)

Sodium carbonate	9	Sodium alkyl sulphate (powder)	1

Method Mix well together and store in a closed container. Perfume oils may be added as desired.

Bath cubes are compressed blocks of this mixture. Starch powder may be added to help binding.

Bath oils and essences

(a)

Isopropyl myristate	$5\frac{1}{4}$	Perfume oil	As desired
Oleyl alcohol	$4\frac{3}{4}$		

122

(b)

Isopropyl myristate	3	Mineral oil	$3\frac{1}{2}$
Diethyl phthalate	1	Perfume oil	As desired

These mixtures may have colour dye added to give them an attractive appearance.

(c)

Triethanolamine oleate	1	Perfume oil	1
Water	98		

(d)

Triethanolamine lauryl		Water	$3\frac{1}{2}$
sulphate	5	Perfume oil	$\frac{1}{2}$

Pine oil is very suitable for using in bath essences.

Bubble baths

Triethanolamine alkyl		Water	5
sulphate	4	Perfume oil	$\frac{1}{2}$
Nonyl phenol			
(condensate)	1		

Method Mix the perfume oil with the nonyl phenol using gentle heat to dissolve. Then add the triethanolamine alkyl sulphate, followed by the water, and blend well.

Note These products may have a cosmetic preservative incorporated. Formaldehyde (40 per cent) is suitable for the purpose used at the rate of not over $\frac{1}{10}$ fluid ounce to each 50 fluid ounces of the main mixture.

Gel

Gelatine	5	Glycerine	11
Sodium lauryl ether		Water	62
sulphate	60	Perfume oil	5

Method Heat the glycerine. Soak the gelatine in the water and mix with the glycerine. Then add the sodium lauryl ether sulphate and the perfume oil. Cool and put in closed jars.

Soaps

Home soap making was an old household industry in former times. Here is a recipe for a simple, rich-lather soap for the face:

Tallow	30	Caustic potash solution	
Coconut oil	18	(Potasssium hydroxide)	12
Stearic acid	$34\frac{3}{4}$	Perfume oil	2
Caustic soda solution			
(Sodium hydroxide)	$5\frac{1}{3}$		

Method Mix ingredients well, using heat, stir vigorously and cool. Fancy shapes may be made by using moulds. To obtain different colours of soap, use cosmetic dyestuffs.

Note Sodium hydroxide and potassium hydroxide may be dissolved at the rate of $3\frac{1}{2}$ ounce to 2 pints or 10 fluid ounces of water to make the caustic soda and castic potash solutions respectively.

Germicidal soap

Castor oil	50	Water	100
Caustic soda	$6\frac{1}{2}$		

Method Heat these ingredients to make the soap. Then add to each 6 ounces of soap: 1 ounce of parachlormetaxylenol, 1 ounce of terpineol, 1 ounce of terpinolene, and some water. Blend well, cool, and leave to set in bars or blocks. Cut into suitable portions for bath use. Perfume, generally pine oil, can be included if you like.

After-bath oil or lotion

Almond oil	8	Olive oil	4
Sunflower oil	12	Wheatgerm or maize oil	4
Groundnut oil	8	Perfume oil, as favoured	$\frac{1}{2}$–1

Method Mix well and keep in closed container.

After-bath moisturizer

Mineral oil	$3\frac{3}{4}$	Propylene glycol	10
Silicone oil	$1\frac{1}{4}$	Glycerine	20
Lanolin	5	Water Enough to form a	
Isopropyl myristate	10	cream of desired consistency	

Method Heat the mineral oil, the silicone oil, the lanolin and the isopropyl myristate together, then heat separately the glycerine and the propylene glycol. Add the second mixture to the first, stir well and start putting in water, mixing continuously, until a stiffish cream is formed. Then add some perfume oil and cool.

Talcum and dusting powders

(a)

Calcium carbonate	25	Talc	70
Zinc stearate	5	Perfume oil	As desired

Method Mix well and sprinkle in perfume oil.

(b)

Magnesium carbonate	15	Talc	75
Zinc stearate	5	Perfume oil	As desired
Zinc oxide	5		

(c) *For after shaving*

Calcium carbonate	8	Suntan cosmetic	
Zinc oxide	4	pigment	As necessary
Talc	88	Perfume oil	As desired

Deodorant powder

Calcium carbonate	5	Bithional	$\frac{1}{2}$
Zinc oxide	10	Talc	$79\frac{1}{2}$
Zinc stearate	5	Perfume oil	As desired

For babies

Rice starch	20	Talc	65
Zinc oxide	15		

Baby powders should not contain boric acid powder. If desired, a light sprinkling of rose perfume oil may be added.

For prickly heat

Calcium carbonate	5	Undecylenic acid	2
Zinc stearate	2	Zinc undecylenate	10
Menthol	$\frac{1}{2}$	Talc	$80\frac{3}{4}$

Talcum powders should always be sieved after mixing and kept in closed containers.

Depilatories

Paste

(a)

Strontium sulphide	15	Glycerine	4
Titanium dioxide	$1\frac{1}{2}$	Gum tragacanth	$2\frac{1}{2}$
Zinc oxide	$3\frac{1}{2}$	Lime water	21
Calcium carbonate	$2\frac{1}{2}$	Perfume oil	$\frac{1}{8}$

Method   Mix the gum tragacanth with part of the glycerine and the water to make a mucilage. Add the zinc oxide and the titanium dioxide bit by bit to the rest of the glycerine, and mix with this. Now add the strontium sulphide, the calcium carbonate, lime water and the perfume oil. Mix well until smooth and well blended.

Use   Spread the paste thinly on the skin over the hair, leave on for about three minutes, and then scrape and wash off.

Note   If any irritation results, remove at once.

Cream

Calcium thioglycollate trihydrate	6	Glycerine	5
Calcium carbonate	20	Water	$61\frac{1}{2}$
Titanium dioxide	2	Pefume oil	As desired
Cetyl alcohol	5	Calcium hydroxide	$\frac{1}{3}$
Sodium lauryl sulphate (powder)	$\frac{1}{2}$		

Method Add the titanium dioxide to the glycerine bit by bit, then melt the cetyl alcohol, and mix it with these and a little of the water. Make separately a mix of the sodium lauryl sulphate, calcium hydroxide, and calcium thioglycollate trihydrate. Add this to the calcium carbonate, already mixed with some of the water. Now blend together these two mixtures. Stir continuously, incorporating the rest of the water, to make a cream.

Note Observe the same precautions as for the paste above.

Waxes

(a)

Beeswax	2	Rosin	7
Ozokerite	1	Perfume oil	As desired

Method Heat and mix, then filter and cool.

(b)

Beeswax	4	Rosin	4
Candelilla wax	$\frac{1}{2}$	Perfume oil	As desired
Isopropyl myristate	$1\frac{1}{2}$		

| Petroleum jelly | $\frac{1}{2}$ | Paraffin wax | $1\frac{7}{8}$ |
| Beeswax | $2\frac{1}{2}$ | Perfume oil | As desired |

Use To apply, first soften the depilatory waxes by gentle heating, then spread them over the hairs on the skin with a suitable brush. When the depilatory has cooled, pull the hairs out. Use this preparation with caution in case it causes skin trouble through continual application.

Foot powders

(a)

| Talc | 100 | Boric acid powder | $1\frac{1}{2}$ |
| Camphor | 1 | | |

(b)

| Starch powder | 95 | Methylditannin | 5 |

(c)

| Starch powder | 20 | Oxyquinoline sulphate | 1 |
| Boric acid powder | 10 | Talc | 69 |

(d)

| Starch powder | 45 | Talc | 45 |
| Boric acid powder | 10 | | |

Method Mix well and store in a closed container. Dust freely on feet, especially between the toes.

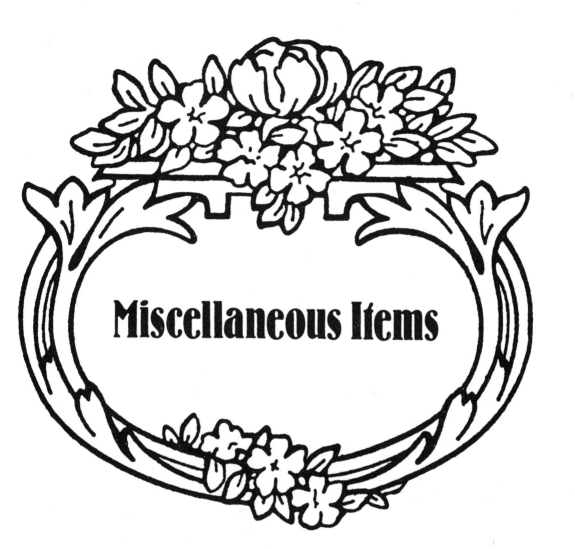

Miscellaneous Items

Shaving materials

Soaps and creams

(a)

Coconut oil	5	Sodium hydroxide	$\frac{3}{4}$
Stearic acid	15	Glycerine	5
Palm kernel oil	$2\frac{1}{2}$	Water	$18\frac{1}{4}$
Potassium hydroxide	$3\frac{1}{2}$	Perfume oil	$\frac{1}{4}$

Method Mix one half of the stearic acid with the coconut and palm kernel oils, put in a double pan and heat. Add the sodium hydroxide, water and glycerine and stir well. When blended, put in the rest of the stearic acid and other ingredients, plus some extra water if necessary, continue stirring, cool, and leave to set.

(b)

Olive oil	2	Potassium hydroxide	$1\frac{1}{2}$
Coconut oil	6	Sodium hydroxide	$\frac{1}{3}$
Glycerine	4	Water	46
Stearic acid	38	Perfume	As required
Lecithin	2		

Method Prepare as for *(a)*, mixing half of the stearic acid with the oils first, and then adding the rest of the materials.

Liquid cream

Coconut oil	$8\frac{1}{2}$	Almond oil	1
Stearic acid	$8\frac{1}{2}$	Alcohol	3
Glycerine	8	Water	$68\frac{3}{4}$
Potassium hydroxide	$2\frac{1}{2}$	Perfume oil	As desired

Method Mix as for the soap creams.

Brushless

(a)

Stearic acid	20	Glycerine	7
Cetyl alcohol	$\frac{1}{2}$	Water	$69\frac{1}{2}$
Mineral oil	2	Perfume oil	As desired
Potassium hydroxide	1		

(b)

Stearic acid	16	Ammonia solution	2
Mineral oil	14	Water	60
Spermaceti	2	Perfume oil	As desired
Glycerine	6		

Method   Melt the stearic acid, spermaceti and mineral oil in a double pan, then add the glycerine and ammonia and finally the water. As the mixture cools add the perfume oil. Stir continuously. Cool and put in closed containers.

Dry shaving

(a) For pre-shaving

Sorbitol	5	Water	49
Lactic acid	1	Perfume oil	As desired
Alcohol	45		

Method   Mix the ingredients well together to make a lotion.

(b)

Talc	5	Colloidal silica	2
Kaolin	1	Chalk	1
Zinc oxide	1		

(c)

Kaolin	5	Talc	88
Zinc			
or magnesium stearate	7		

Aftershave

Lotions

(a)

Glycerine	3	Witchhazel	$84\frac{3}{4}$
Boric acid	2	Perfume oil	As desired
Menthol	$\frac{1}{10}$		

(b)

Glycerine	5	Bay rum	94
Peppermint oil	1	Perfume oil	As desired

(c)

Glycerine	15	Alcohol	40
Menthol	$\frac{1}{2}$	Water	$56\frac{3}{4}$
Cetrimide	$\frac{1}{2}$	Perfume oil	As desired

Cream type

Mineral oil	4	Menthol	$\frac{1}{10}$
Glyceryl monostearate	15	Alcohol	5
Glycerine	6	Water	$68\frac{7}{8}$
Boric acid	1	Perfume oil	As desired

Method Dissolve the menthol and the perfume oil in the

134

alcohol and add to the other ingredients, which should have been previously heated in a double pan. Stir well, cool, and store.

Powder

Talc	$8\frac{1}{2}$	Perfume oil	As desired
Boric acid	$\frac{1}{5}$	Colour	Enough to give a
Magnesium stearate	1	flesh or a tinted suntan look	

Method   Mix well and store in a dry container. This powder should not be overperfumed.

Manicure preparations

Cuticle creams

Beeswax	1	Petroleum jelly	95
Lanolin, anhydrous	4	Perfume oil	As desired

Method   Mix well and put in a closed container.

Cuticle remover

Glycerine	25	Water	73
Potassium hydroxide	2	Perfume oil	As desired

Stain removers and nail bleach

(a)

Paraffin wax	$2\frac{1}{2}$	Borax	$\frac{1}{4}$
Beeswax	5	Water	15
Mineral oil	23	Perfume oil	$\frac{1}{8}$
Pumicestone powder	4		

Method   Mix the borax with the water and heat. Add this to the mineral oil and waxes. Drop the pumice in slowly bit by bit and mix to a thick cream. Stir continuously, cool and store.

(b)

Glycerine	10	Water	$89\frac{1}{2}$
Hydrochloric acid	$\frac{1}{4}$		

(c)

Citric or tartaric acid	5	Water	95

(d)

Hydrogen peroxide		Benzoic acid	5 drops
solution	5	Water	$3\frac{7}{8}$
Glycerine	1		

Method   Mix well and store in closed containers.

Nail polishes
Abrasive

Stannic oxide	45	Colour and perfume	
Powdered silica	4		As desired
Butyl stearate	1		

Method   Mix well and use. If a paste is wanted, moisten with a little glycerine.

Wax polish

Hardened palm		Synthetic wax	$3\frac{1}{2}$
kernel oil	11	Stannic oxide	$30\frac{1}{2}$

Other materials, such as beeswax, ceresine, petroleum jelly or rosin may be used.

Nail white

This gives an even white edge to the nails.

Cream

Petroleum jelly	31	Titanium dioxide	19

Method   Mix well and use.

Wax

Beeswax	$27\frac{1}{2}$	Lanolin	$4\frac{1}{2}$
Cocoa butter	$4\frac{1}{2}$	Cotton seed oil	$4\frac{1}{2}$
Castor oil	4	Titanium dioxide	5

Method   A little gum arabic, made into a mucilage with hot water, can be added to bind the materials. Mix and leave to set.

To treat brittle nails

Cream

White petroleum jelly	$7\frac{1}{2}$	Triethanolamine	5
White beeswax	$2\frac{1}{2}$	Glycerine	6
Lanolin	$2\frac{1}{2}$	Water	$31\frac{1}{2}$

Method   Heat the white petroleum jelly, the white beeswax and the lanolin in a double pan, then add the glycerine and the triethanolamine, followed by the water, stirring continuously. Mix well and allow to cool. Store in a closed container.

Strengthener or hardener

Aluminium chloride	5	Soft soap	1
Glycerine	10	Alcohol	5
Formaldehyde		Water	$78\frac{3}{4}$
(40 per cent)	$\frac{1}{10}$		

Method Mix the aluminium chloride, the glycerine and the soft soap in the water, using heat. Add the alcohol and the formaldehyde, blending well.

Both the above recipes may have some perfume oil included.

Baby preparations

Baby oil

(a)

White mineral oil	49	Lanolin	$\frac{1}{2}$

(b)

Groundnut oil	27	White mineral oil	$22\frac{1}{2}$

Baby lotion

Lanolin	$3\frac{1}{4}$	Maize oil	$1\frac{1}{2}$
Petroleum jelly	2	Propylene glycol	10
Sesame oil	$1\frac{1}{2}$	Water	$20\frac{1}{3}$

Method Mix the oils first, heating slowly, then add the water and stir until well blended.

Baby cream

Lanolin	1	Petroleum jelly	2
Beeswax or other		White mineral oil	2
soft wax	$7\frac{1}{2}$	Water	$37\frac{1}{2}$

Method Mix well and use.

Setting lotion for babies' hair

Glycerine	7	Water	$42\frac{1}{2}$
Gum tragacanth	$\frac{1}{2}$		

Method Dissolve the gum in the water by heating and then add the glycerine, mixing well.

Note Small amounts of perfume oil may be added to the above listed preparations. Rose oil is quite suitable.

Skin lightening

These preparations are intended to lighten the natural skin colour or for the treatment of freckles.

Bleaching cream

Mineral oil	3	Hydroquinone	2
Cetyl alcohol	10	Glycerine	5
Sodium lauryl sulphate	$1\frac{1}{2}$	Ascorbic acid	$\frac{1}{2}$
Potassium		Water	$77\frac{3}{4}$
metabisulphite	$\frac{1}{10}$	Perfume oil	$\frac{1}{4}$

Method   Dissolve the hydroquinone, the potassium meta-bisulphite and the sodium lauryl sulphate in the water. Then add the glycerine and the ascorbic acid, heat and stir gently. Now put this mixture into another pan containing the mineral oil and the cetyl alcohol, which should have been previously warmed and mixed. Blend well, stirring continuously, and add the perfume oil while cooling.

Note   Preservatives may be added.

It is important when preparing this bleaching cream to use stainless steel pans. Do not let the hydroquinone fall on your skin. Skin lightener should not be used by anyone whose skin reacts unfavourably to the preparation.

Some shop-sold bleaching creams may contain ammoniated mercury which is absorbed by the skin and is poisonous. This substance should not be used.

Health salts

Cream of tartar	6	Bicarbonate of soda	6
Tartaric acid	6		

Method   Mix well together, and add:

Powdered magnesia	3	Magnesium sulphate	6

Blend well and store in a closed jar. To sweeten the health salts use a little saccharin. The tablets can be crushed up and added to suit individual taste.

Use   One teaspoonful to a glass of lukewarm water.

140

Hand cleansers

(a)

Soap flakes	30	Lanolin	5
Bentonite	30	Perfume oil	1
Detergent	10	Water	24

Method   Mix the bentonite and the detergent together, then heat the soap flakes and lanolin gently with the water. Add the first mixture to this, stir well and add perfume. When fully blended, cool and store.

(b)

Sulphonated castor oil	$47\frac{1}{2}$	Detergent	1
Castor oil	$\frac{1}{2}$		

Method   Mix and use.

(c)

Sulphonated castor oil	$22\frac{1}{2}$	Maize or oatmeal	50
Butyl stearate	$22\frac{1}{2}$	(medium ground)	
Oleic acid	5		

Mix the first three ingredients together and then add the meal. Fine sawdust may be used instead of meal, especially pine sawdust.

(d)

Powdered soap	50	Borax	2
Fine sawdust	48		

Method   Mix well and use.

Protective or barrier cream

Paraffin wax	12	Water	70
Glyceryl monostearate	12	Perfume oil	$\frac{1}{4}$
Lanolin	6		

Method   Heat the first three ingredients, stir well and then add the water. While cooling, add the perfume oil.

Acne treatment

Borax	10	Methyl salicylate	$\frac{1}{10}$
Sodium bicarbonate	5	Alcohol	$12\frac{1}{2}$
Menthol	$\frac{1}{10}$	Glycerine	50
Thymol	$\frac{1}{10}$	Water	422
Talc or kieselguhr	As required		

Method   Dissolve the borax and the sodium bicarbonate in the water, then add the glycerine. The methyl salicylate, the menthol and the thymol should be dissolved in the alcohol. Now combine the two mixtures and add to them enough talc or kieselguhr to make a lotion. When well blended, store in a closed container.

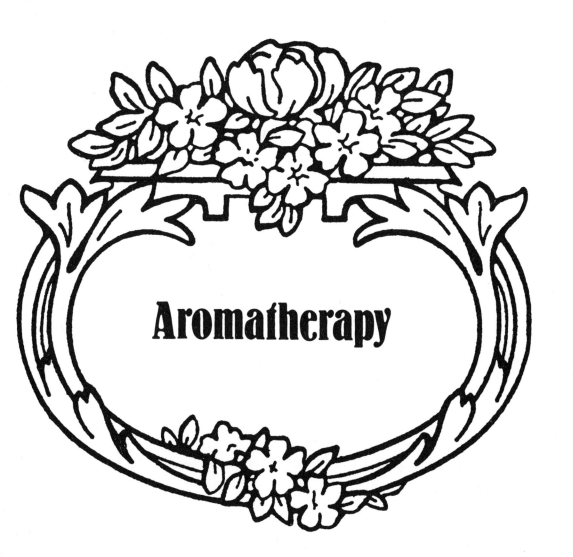

Aromatherapy

Aromatherapy is the use of aromatic essences, oils or extracts from plants for the treatment and alleviation of various body conditions. The treatment is usually carried out in conjunction with massage, bathing or similar exercises. The pleasant smell and stimulating effects of the materials have a powerful influence on mental and physical wellbeing.

A major advantage of aromatherapy is that it can be practised cheaply and easily, without inconvenience or lengthy treatment sessions. Many people cannot manage to attend time-consuming expensive recuperative courses, or stay at health centres. But simple aromatic oil therapy may be undertaken at home, or, if more advanced massages are desired, at clinics. More relaxation can be obtained after an hour's treatment with essential oils than most people can achieve during a weekend or more of exercises or patent diets. There is nothing secretive, or weird, about aromatherapy; it is quick and straightforward to use and only natural, freely available plant oils are needed.

Aromatherapy is curative and preventive. The relaxation produced by the essential oils when they are massaged into the skin helps recuperation from run-down conditions. Rejuvenation is aided, too. Other effects include a high degree of energy increase, with rises in mental and physical vitality, and consequent general build-up of resistance to tension and strain. This helps to discourage headaches and stops worrying and irritability, producing confidence and assurance at work and in social life. Men, in particular, are sensitive to prolonged tension and suffer in the spinal region. The soothing results of essential oil application can aid greatly in relieving such troubles. Women also find aromatherapy valuable to reduce nervous strain. Many essential oils are excellent for stopping acne, spots, and pimples, or for treating burns and healing scars. Insomnia, rheumatic conditions and muscular contractions can also be helped by aromatic oil therapy. Some continental doctors and surgeons use the methods to strengthen muscles and skin tissue before operations, as well as to remove scars afterwards.

Using essential oils

Only small quantities of essential oils are employed in aromatherapy. It is not necessary to buy more than an ounce or two at any one time, so concentrated are the essences. The finger-tips should be immersed in the oils, then massaged gently over the skin. Rubbing is undesirable, but soothing and relaxing therapy is obtained by running the fingers lightly along the length of the back and around the head. This should continue for periods of up to an hour, with intervals every ten minutes or so to allow the oils to exercise their recuperative and stimulating effects. Before the end of this time, body and mind feel invigorated and relaxed.

There is a wide choice of oils for aromatic therapy. Different types are beneficial for various kinds of people, and account should be taken of the particular perfumes that are liked by individuals. Oils like rose, geranium, basil, lavender, bay, lime, lemon or orange, patchouli and sandalwood are highly scented.

Thyme, marjoram, sage, mint, pine and eucalyptus have germicidal odours. Dill, fennel, coriander, rue, calamus and balsam have medicinal properties. Rosemary is employed in the manufacture of Eau de Cologne.

Plant extracts

Plant extracts are often referred to in cosmetic trade circles as botanicals. For a long time manuals of health and beauty have given extensive lists of fruits, nuts, garden plants, tree and shrub barks, mosses, roots and rhizomes or tubers, seeds, flowers and bulbs that produce useful treatments for various complaints or problems.

Freckle lotion

Angelica	5	Styrax	2
Black bellebore root	5	Water	88

Method Cut up the solid ingredients and soak them in the water for two to three weeks. Strain and bottle.

Use Apply to freckles several times daily.

Skin cleanser

A good skin cleanser can be prepared by mixing 10 parts of sweet almond oil with 10 parts of bitter almond oil and adding 1 part of powdered hard soap. (All these parts are measured by volume, not by weight.) Heat and blend well, then store in a closed container.

Antiperspirant-deodorant

Tincture of arnica	5	Witchhazel	92
Glycerol	3		

Keep in a stoppered bottle.

Anti-wrinkle pomade

| Lily bulb juice | 6 | White beeswax | 3 |
| Honey | $1\frac{1}{2}$ | Rosewater | $1\frac{1}{4}$ |

Use heat to mix well and apply at night.

The juices of strawberries, lilies, jasmine, lettuce, milkweed and dandelions are also said to have beneficial effects on the skin. The tubers of water-lilies and cucumbers produce juices that are useful skin toners.

To get a better idea of the effects of the extracts of some different plants on the skin we can group them as follows:

Astringent (binding or contracting the skin) – witchhazel, hazelnut, cornflower, rose, clover, plantain, geranium, myrtle, cypress, rhatany.

Tranquillizing (soothing the skin) – orange flower, mallow, linden, cherry laurel, pepitgrain.

Healing – lavender, cornflower, sage.

Toning – witchhazel, rose, elderberry.

Emollient (softening) – lettuce, mallow, ylang-ylang, althea, Iceland moss, fenugreek, salep.

Rubefacient (reddening of skin) – juniper, arnica, pine, rosemary, capsicum, nasturtium, bryony.

Decongestant and lenitive (clearing away and easing pain) – camomile, peppermint, sweet almond, linden.

Antiseptic – echinacea (rattlesnake weed).

Balsamic (producing balsam, healing effects) – anise, melissa, orange, rose, cinnamon, lemon.

Emollient lotions   One of the oldest cosmetic lotions for soothing the skin was made from milk of almonds, honey and rosewater. The procedure is to take some almonds, blanch them with a little boiling water, and squash them up and strain to make a 'milk'. To this milk of almonds is added some honey and enough rosewater to produce a well-blended lotion. Another formula reads:

Blanched almonds	$12\frac{1}{2}$	Borax	$\frac{3}{4}$
Beeswax	$\frac{7}{8}$	Alcohol	$1\frac{1}{4}$
Spermaceti	$\frac{3}{4}$	Bitter almond water	65
Hard powdered soap	$\frac{3}{4}$		

Method   Mix well together and add a little almond oil, if liked. Bitter almond water is made by blanching the almonds and then squashing and straining to give a liquid. Dilute with plain water as required.

Parsley, ginseng, alfalfa (lucerne), and watercress extracts are also said to have cosmetic value. Among fruits, apricots, avocados, peaches and papayas are used for beautifying or related purposes. Chlorophyll, the green colouring matter found in plants, is a popular preventive of objectionable odours.

148

Plants used in making cosmetics

Bark or wood Oak, hazel, cinchona, witchhazel, birch, quillaia, poplar.

Flowers Lupin, rose, arnica, elder, linden, calendula, hawthorn, saffron, cloves, camomile, melissa, eupatorium, cornflower, jasmine, violet, St John's Wort, aletris, mallow, yarrow.

Fruits Avocado, banana, tomato, cucumber, strawberry, raspberry, currants, myrtle, pumpkin, pineapple, lemon, lime, orange, grapefruit, fig, apricot, blueberry, cherry, grape, peach, pear, plum, colocynth, blackberry, papaya, whortleberry.

Leaves Nettle, witchhazel, spinach, lettuce, celery, althea, plantain, alfalfa, watercress, parsley, peppermint, aloe, rosemary, eucalyptus, birch, bay, pine needles, mullein, cherry laurel, pilocarpus, thyme, sage, bryony, cactus, agaves, clover, olive, milkweed, spearmint.

Mosses Iceland moss, Irish moss, kelp.

Nuts Almonds, hazel or cob (filbert), pistachio.

Roots Burdock, orris, althea, licorice, valerian, tormentilla, angelica, nettle, black hellebore, dandelion, carrot, comfrey, ginseng, saponaria.

Seeds Peas, lentils, wheatgerm, maize germ, barley germ, oats, coriander, nutmeg, linseed, quince, psyllium, wheat (including wheat bran).

149

Resins and oleo-resins Benzoin, balsam of Peru, myrrh, storax or styrax, tolu.

Tubers and bulbs Lily, onion, wild onion, garlic.

Miscellaneous Cantharides, birch sap, Venice turpentine, Austrian turpentine, cochineal, carthamus, chlorophyll, carotene, catechu, cudbear, caramel, alkanet, indigo, annatto, yeast, red sandalwood, mistletoe, lappa, equisetum, chlorella, corn silk, hay, saponine.

For a list of essential oils please see Appendix D.

150

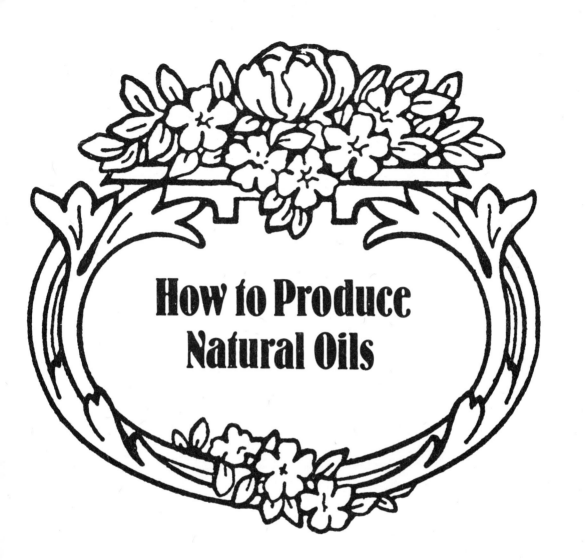

How to Produce
Natural Oils

There are a number of different methods of producing natural plant oils, including pressing, maceration, enfleurage, expression and distillation. Some of these are not suitable for the home producer because they require complicated equipment, but it is not difficult to distil or macerate your own essential oils at home, using plants grown in your garden.

Cultivation

The cultivation of herbs and scented plants is popular today. Essential oils can be extracted from a wide range of plants. Lavender, rose geranium, balm, peppermint, basil, sage, thyme, verbena, valerian, camomile, roses, rosemary, spike lavender and others are quite straightforward to grow.

Well known and reliable suppliers include:

Thompson & Morgan Ltd.,
London Road, Ipswich, Suffolk, England, U.K.

Samuel Dobie & Son Ltd.,
Upper Dee Mills,
Llangollen, Clwyd, Wales, U.K.

Vilmorin-Andrieux et Cie,
La Menitre,
49250 Beaufort-en-Vallée, France.

Distillation

Simple-pattern stills can be heated by gas or paraffin burners. The plant material is placed in the boiler on top of the grid and as the steam from the boiling water passes through it, the fragrant oils are carried up the gooseneck with the vapour and into the condenser. They pass through this and trickle out into the separator and are finally collected.

Material for distilling should be collected from the plants in the morning, as early as possible but after any dew has evaporated from the leaves. It may consist of flowers, leaves and stalks, either singly or combined or sometimes the whole plants. Leave the plants for an hour or two to wilt and then pack the material evenly in the still. See that it is evenly distributed inside, and not too loose in one place and too tight in another, otherwise the steam will not pass satisfactorily through it. Close the still door and light the heater. When the water boils the steam will begin to move through the plant material and carry off the oil and water vapour. As these pass through the condenser they cool and run off as liquid into the separator. Continue distillation until no more oil comes off. You may have to add more water during the operation. Never let the still run dry. Distillation may take from one to three hours depending upon the type of plant material.

When finished, pour the oil gently out of the separator into bottles and put on stoppers. Store to mature. The water in the still can be strained and, if you like, used for cosmetic or toilet purposes.

Dry weather produces the best quality and highest yields of ethereal oils. Test the plants for condition by breaking off a tiny portion, squeezing it between the thumb and fore-finger and smelling the broken tissue to find out the strength and scent of the oil present. Normally mature plants are the highest-yielding ones. With perennials, several cuttings or harvests can be obtained at intervals.

A reliable supplier of stills is Baird & Tatlock Ltd (address in List of Suppliers).

153

Maceration

Immerse the plant material, normally flowers, in hot oil or fat (odourless vegetable grease or refined lard or beef suet), at a temperature of 140°–158°F (60°–70°C) in a pan or other vessel. Stir continuously and when the scent oil has passed from the material into the fat, usually after about half an hour, pour the hot contents of the pan through a sieve into another pot. Discard the material left on the sieve and return the scented liquified fat to the first pan, to be filled with a fresh lot of flowers. Repeat the process several times until the fragrance of the concentrated scented grease is strong and satisfactory. Finally, pour the hot scented fat into pots to cool.

Boiling

Put the plant material into pots of boiling water and keep it there until all the oil has passed into the water, which takes half to three-quarters of an hour. It is important always to keep the material under the boiling water, because if it touches the hot, dry sides of the pot it will produce a nasty smell. Then place the whole mass on a sieve and let the liquid collect in another vessel. Discard the exhausted plant material. When the liquid cools, the oil will separate from the water, rising to the top, and can be gently poured off.

Pressing

In this method the plant material is crushed in a powerful press or between rollers, and the extracted oil runs down and collects in a tray. Oil seeds are also treated in this way. The method is generally used for obtaining oil from the peels of oranges and other citrus fruits.

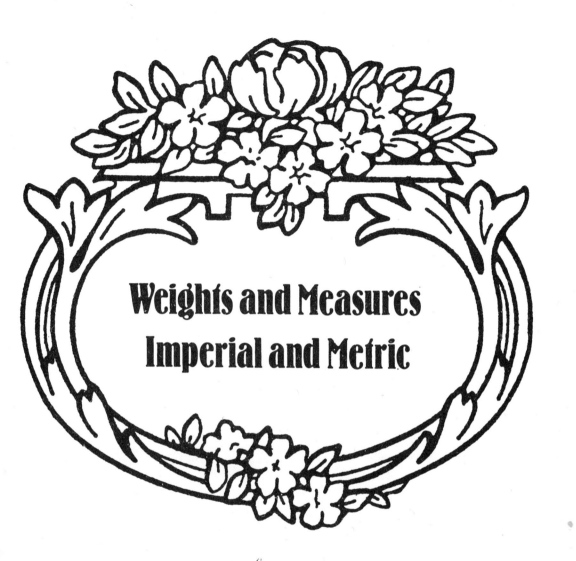

Weights and Measures
Imperial and Metric

Imperial system

Avoirdupois dry measure

$$27{\cdot}34375 \text{ grains} = 1 \text{ dram}$$
$$16 \text{ drams} = 1 \text{ ounce}$$
$$437{\cdot}5 \text{ grains} = 1 \text{ ounce}$$
$$16 \text{ ounces} = 1 \text{ lb}$$
$$7000 \text{ grains} = 1 \text{ lb}$$

1 dram $= \frac{1}{16}$ ounce		$\frac{1}{8}$ ounce $=$ 2 drams	
$\frac{1}{2}$ dram $= \frac{1}{32}$ ounce		$\frac{1}{4}$ ounce $=$ 4 drams	
$\frac{1}{4}$ dram $= \frac{1}{64}$ ounce		$\frac{1}{2}$ ounce $=$ 8 drams	
$\frac{1}{8}$ dram $= \frac{1}{128}$ ounce		$\frac{3}{4}$ ounce $=$ 12 drams	

Apothecaries' fluid measure

$$60 \text{ minims} = 1 \text{ fluid drachm}$$
$$8 \text{ fluid drachms} = 1 \text{ fluid ounce}$$
$$480 \text{ minims} = 1 \text{ fluid ounce}$$
$$20 \text{ fluid ounces} = 1 \text{ pint}$$
$$9{,}600 \text{ minims} = 1 \text{ pint}$$

1 fluid ounce $=$ 437·5 grains (weight of this measure of distilled water at 62° F)

1 ounce avoirdupois $=$ 1 fluid ounce in weight (437·5 grains, based on quantity of distilled water at 62°F)

Equivalents in metric system

Dry measures

1 grain	=	0·0648 gramme
1 dram	=	1·772 grammes
1 ounce	=	28·350 grammes
1 lb (16 ounces or 7000 grains)	=	0·45359243 kilogramme
1 milligramme	=	0·015 grain
1 centigramme	=	0·154 grain
1 decigramme	=	1·543 grains
1 gramme	=	15·432 grains
1 dekagramme	=	5·644 drams
1 hectogramme	=	3·527 ounces
1 kilogramme (1000 grammes)	=	2·2046223 lb

Fluid measures

1 minim	=	0·059 millilitre
1 fluid drachm (60 minims)	=	3·552 millilitres
1 fluid ounce (8 fluid drachms)	=	2·84123 centilitres
1 pint (20 fluid ounces)	=	0·568 litre
1 gallon	=	4·546 litres
1 millilitre	=	1 cubic centimetre
1 centilitre	=	10 cubic centimetres
1 litre	=	1000 cubic centimetres (cc)

Common equivalents

Liquids

1 teaspoonful	=	60 drops
		60 minims
		1 fluid drachm
		4 cubic centimetres
1 drop	=	1 minim
1 thimbleful	=	30 drops or 30 minims or $\frac{1}{2}$ fluid drachm (ie $\frac{1}{16}$ fluid ounce)
1 dessertspoonful	=	2 fluid drachms or $\frac{1}{4}$ fluid ounce
1 tablespoonful	=	4 fluid drachms or $\frac{1}{2}$ fluid ounce
2 tablespoonfuls	=	1 fluid ounce
10 tablespoonfuls	=	$\frac{1}{4}$ pint
1 wineglassful	=	$2\frac{1}{4}$ fluid ounces
1 teacupful	=	5 fluid ounces
1 breakfastcupful	=	8 fluid ounces
1 tumblerful	=	from 10 to 12 fluid ounces

(Cups and tumblers should be of recognized standard sizes)

Dry materials

1 rounded saltspoonful	=	$\frac{1}{8}$ ounce
1 rounded teaspoonful	=	$\frac{1}{4}$ ounce
1 level dessertspoonful	=	$\frac{1}{4}$ ounce
1 rounded dessertspoonful	=	$\frac{1}{2}$ ounce
1 level tablespoonful	=	$\frac{1}{2}$ ounce
1 rounded tablespoonful	=	1 ounce
1 teacupful	=	6 ounces
1 breakfastcupful	=	8 ounces

Fats

A portion the size of a small egg weighs on average 1 ounce

1 level teacupful = 8 ounces

158

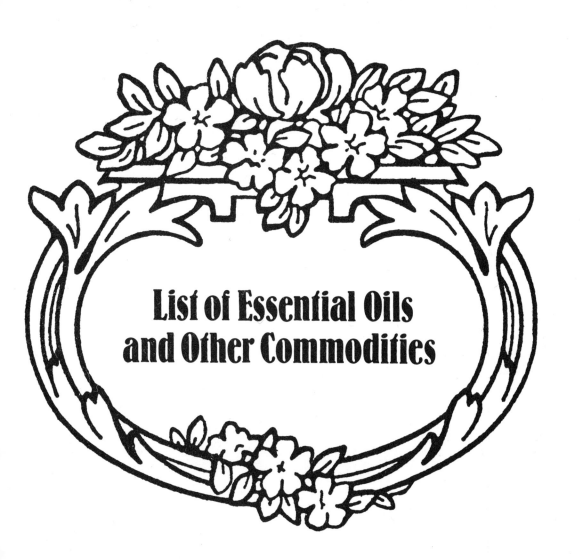

List of Essential Oils
and Other Commodities

Note This list is not intended to be an exhaustive one.

Essential Oils

Almond, bitter	Citronella	Litsea Cubeba
Ambrette seed	Clary sage	Lovage
Aniseed pimpinella	Clove bud	Mandarin
Aniseed (star)	Clove leaf	Myrrh
Asafoetida	Copaiba	Neroli
Basil	Coriander	Nutmeg
Bay	Costus	Olibanum
Bergamot	Cubeb	Onion
Birch	Cumin	Opoponax
Birch tar	Cypress	Orange, bitter
Bois de rose	Dill	Orange, sweet
Buchu	Elemi	Origanum
Cade	Eucalyptus	Orris
Cajuput	Fennel	Palmarosa
Calamus	Galbanum	Parsley
Camomile	Geranium	Patchouli
Camphor white	Ginger	Pennyroyal
Cananga	Gingergrass	Pepper
Caraway	Grapefruit	Peppermint
Cardamon	Guaiacwood	Peru balsam
Carrot seed	Ho	Petitgrain
Cascarilla	Hyssop	Pimento berry
Cassia	Juniper Berry	Pine
Cedarwood	Lavandin	Rosemary
Celery	Lavender	Rose otto
Cinnamon bark	Lemon	Rue
Cinnamon leaf	Lemon grass	Sage
Ciste	Lime	Sandalwood

Sassafras	Tea-tree	Vetivert
Shiu	Thyme	Wintergreen
Spearmint	Turpentine	Wormwood
Spike lavender	Valerian	Ylang-ylang
Tarragon	Verbena	

Floral absolutes and concretes

Ambrette	Jasmine	Rosemary
Boronia	Jonquil	Tuberose
Carnation	Lavandin	Verbena
Cassie	Lavender	Violet leaves
Clary sage	Mimosa	
Genet (broom)	Narcissus	
Immortelle	Orange flower	
(everlasting)	Rose de mai	

Resinoids

Benzoin	Iris	Patchouli
Castoreum	Labdanum (ciste)	Peru
Civet	Mastic	Pine moss
Clove buds	Myrrh	Styrax
Costus	Oak moss	Tolu
Elemi	Olibanum	Tonka beans
Galbanum	Opoponax	Vanilla

Fats and oils

Fatty acids

Capric acid	Myristic acid	Split palm oil
Coconut oil	Palm oil	Split palm kernel
Distilled dehydrated	Palm kernel oil	oil
castor oil	Palmitic acid	Stearic acid
Groundnut or	Ricinollic	Tallow
peanut oil	Soft mixed acid oil	Tobacco seed oil
Lanolin	Soya bean oil	Vegetable oil
Lauric acid	Soya acid oil	
Linseed oil	Split castor oil	

Fixed oils

Almond oil	Corn oil	Sesame oil
(expressed)	Cottonseed oil	Sunflower seed oil
Avocado oil	Olive oil	Tea seed oil
Castor oil	Palm oil	
Coconut oil	Palm kernel oil	Oleine (Oleic Acid)
Cocoa butter	Rape seed oil	Stearine

Gums and thickening agents

Acacia gum	Benzoin	Copal
Agar agar	Canada balsam	Damar
Arabic gum	Carragheen	Galbanum
Asafoetida	Carob bean gum	Guaicum
Bentonite	Copaiba balsam	Karaya gum

162

Myrrh   Psylline seed   Tragacanth gum
Olibanum   Quince seed   Tolu balsam
Pectin   Sandarac
Peru balsam   Shellac

Waxes

Beeswax   Carnauba   Japan wax
Candelilla   Ceresine   Spermaceti

Various

Ambergris   Magnesium carbonate
Ammonium hydroxide   Magnesium stearate
Calamine   Magnesium sulphate
Calcium carbonate   Monoethanolamine
Calcium stearate   Menthol
Cinnamic acid   Musk pods
Citric acid   Paraffin, liquid
Dextrose monohydrate   Petroleum jelly
Diethanolamine   Potassium carbonate
Diglycol laurate   Potassium hydroxide
Glycerine   Salicylic acid
Glyceryl monostearate   Sodium carbonate
Hydrogen peroxide   Sodium hydroxide
Isopropyl myristate   Sodium lauryl sulphate
Kaolin   Sulphur
Kieselguhr   Talc
Lanolin   Tartaric acid
Lecithin   Titanium dioxide

163

Triethanolamine
Triethanolamine lauryl
  sulphate
White mineral oils

Wool alcohols
Zinc oxide
Zinc stearate

Preservatives and antioxidants

Benzoic acid
Boric acid or borax
Methyl parahydroxybenzoate
Potassium sorbate
Propyl parahydroxybenzoate

Sodium benzeate
Sorbic acid
Naphthalene
Rosin
Trisodium phosphate

Solvents

Ethyl alcohol
Methylated spirit
Isopropyl alcohol

Acetone
Propylene glycol
Diethylene glycol

List of Suppliers

Various items may be bought or ordered from retail chemists and pharmacies, druggists, wholesale chemists, health stores, supermarkets and grocers, as well as other shops and merchants.

A list of addresses of the firms given below begins on page 202.

ACETANILIDE
Bush Boake Allen Ltd.,
 Perfumery Division

ACETOGLYCERIDES
Bush Boake Allen Ltd.,
 Perfumery Division

ACETONE
British Celanese Ltd.
The General Chemical Co.,
 Ltd.
Imperial Chemical Industries
 Ltd.
May & Baker Ltd.
Methylating Co. Ltd.
Millwards Merchandise Ltd.
Shell Chemical U.K. Ltd.
J. M. Steel & Co., Ltd.

ACID (ACETIC)
Berk Ltd.
Victor Blagden & Co., Ltd.
British Anhydrous Ammonia
 Co. Ltd.
The General Chemical Co.,
 Ltd.
Hoechst Chemicals Ltd.
Keegan Dyestuffs &
 Chemicals Ltd.
May & Baker Ltd.
Sherman Chemicals Ltd.
Tar Residuals Ltd.

ACID (ADIPIC)
Victor Blagden & Co., Ltd.
Rex Campbell & Co., Ltd.
Dragoco (Gt. Britain) Ltd.
R. W. Greeff & Co. Ltd.
Imperial Chemical Industries
 Ltd.

ACID (BEHENIC)
Armour Hess Chemicals Ltd.
Cyclo Chemicals Ltd.
E. J. R. Lovelock
The Universal Oil Co., Ltd.

ACID (BENZOIC)
Bush Boake Allen Ltd.,
 Perfumery Division
The General Chemical Co.,
 Ltd.
Monsanto Chemicals Ltd.
'Naarden' (London) Ltd.
L. R. B. Pearce Ltd.

ACID (BORIC)
Borax Consolidated, Ltd.
The General Chemical Co.,
 Ltd.
Thomas Morson & Son, Ltd.
Patent Borax Co., Ltd.

ACID (CAPRIC)
Armour Hess Chemicals Ltd.
Cyclo Chemicals Ltd.
E. J. R. Lovelock
Price's (Bromborough) Ltd.
The Universal Oil Co., Ltd.
Wynmouth Lehr & Fatoils
 Ltd.

ACID (CAPRYLIC)
Armour Hess Chemicals Ltd.
Victor Blagden & Co., Ltd.
Cyclo Chemicals Ltd.
E. J. R. Lovelock
Price's (Bromborough) Ltd.
The Universal Oil Co., Ltd.
Wynmouth Lehr & Fatoils
 Ltd.

ACID (CARBOLIC)
See **Phenol**

ACID (CITRIC)
H. J. Evans & Co., Ltd.
F. Gutkind & Co. Ltd.
Kingsley & Keith (Chemicals)
 Ltd.
Millwards Merchandise Ltd.
Pfizer Ltd.
Thomas Morson & Son, Ltd.

Shearman & Co., Ltd.
John & E. Sturge Ltd.

ACID (CRESYLIC)
Anglo-Scottish Chemical Co.
 Ltd.
Victor Blagden & Co. Ltd.
James Greenshields & Co.
 Ltd.
London Tar & Chemicals Co.,
 Ltd.
Midland Tar Distillers Ltd.
Mirvale Chemical Co., Ltd.
Scottish Tar Distillers Ltd.
Tar Residuals Ltd.

ACID (ERUCIC)
Armour Hess Chemicals Ltd.
E. J. R. Lovelock
The Universal Oil Co., Ltd.
Wynmouth Lehr & Fatoils
 Ltd.

ACID (FUMARIC)
Victor Blagden & Co., Ltd.
Bowmans Chemicals Ltd.
Kingsley & Keith (Chemicals)
 Ltd.
Monsanto Chemicals Ltd.

ACID (HYDROCHLORIC)
Barter Trading Corporation
 Ltd.
Berk Spencer Acids Ltd.
W. Blythe & Co., Ltd.
British Anhydrous Ammonia
 Co., Ltd.
Coalite & Chemical Products
 Ltd.
The General Chemical Co.,
 Ltd.
Imperial Chemical Industries
 Ltd.
Laporte Industries (General
 Chemicals Division–Leeds)
Sherman Chemicals Ltd.

166

ACID (LACTIC)
Bowmans Chemical Ltd.
Howards of Ilford Ltd.
Thomas Morson & Son Ltd.
L. R. B. Pearcie Ltd.
P. T. Petley & Co., Ltd.

ACID (LAURIC)
Armour Hess Chemicals Ltd.
Cyclo Chemicals Ltd.
E. J. R. Lovelock
Price's (Bromborough) Ltd.
The Universal Oil Co., Ltd.
Wynmouth Lehr & Fatoils
  Ltd.

ACID (MALIC)
Victor Blagden & Co., Ltd.
Bowmans Chemicals Ltd.

ACID (MYRISTIC)
Armour Hess Chemicals Ltd.
Cyclo Chemicals Ltd.
E. J. R. Lovelock
Price's (Bromborough) Ltd.
The Universal Oil Co., Ltd.
Wynmouth Lehr & Fatoils
  Ltd.

ACID (NITRIC)
Frederick Allen & Sons
  (Chemicals), Ltd.
Berk Ltd.
Berk Spencer Acids Ltd.
The General Chemical Co.,
  Ltd.
Imperial Chemical Industries
  Ltd.
Laporte Industries Ltd.
  (General Chemicals
  Division–Leeds)
Sherman Chemicals Ltd.

ACID (OXALIC)
Frederick Allen & Sons
  (Chemicals), Ltd.
Victor Blagden & Co., Ltd.
Fine Dyestuffs & Chemicals
  Ltd.
The General Chemical Co.,
  Ltd.
Imperial Chemical Industries
  Ltd.
Jessop & Co.
Millwards Merchandise Ltd.
L. R. B. Pearce Ltd.
Thew Arnott & Co., Ltd.
Wynmouth Lehr & Fatoils
  Ltd.

ACID (PALMITIC)
Armour Hess Chemicals Ltd.
Cyclo Chemicals Ltd.
E. J. R. Lovelock
Price's (Bromborough) Ltd.
The Universal Oil Co., Ltd.

ACID (PERACETIC)
Keegan Dyestuffs &
  Chemicals Ltd.
Kingsley & Keith (Chemicals)
  Ltd.
Laporte Industries Ltd.
  (General Chemicals
  Division–Luton)

ACID (PROPIONIC)
Victor Blagden & Co., Ltd.
Distillers Chemicals & Plastics
  Ltd.
Kingsley & Keith (Chemicals)
  Ltd.

ACID (RICINOLEIC)
E. J. R. Lovelock
Price's (Bromborough) Ltd.
The Universal Oil Co., Ltd.

ACID (SALICYLIC)
Bush Boake Allen Ltd.,
  Perfumery Division
H. J. Evans & Co., Ltd.
The General Chemical Co.,
  Ltd.
R. W. Greeff & Co., Ltd.
Kingsley & Keith (Chemicals)
  Ltd.
Monsanto Chemicals Ltd.

ACID (SULPHURIC)
Alwitt Ltd.
Berk Ltd.
W. Blythe & Co., Ltd.
The General Chemical Co.,
  Ltd.
Hardman & Holden Ltd.
Imperial Chemical Industries
  Ltd.
Imperial Smelting
  Corporation (N.S.C.) Ltd.
Laporte Industries Ltd.
  (General Chemicals
  Division–Leeds & Widnes)
London Tar & Chemical Co.,
  Ltd.
Marchon Products Ltd.
Sherman Chemicals Ltd.
Peter Spence & Sons, Ltd.
Staveley Chemicals Ltd.

ACID (TANNIC)
Millwards Merchandise Ltd.

ACID (TARTARIC)
F. Gutkind & Co., Ltd.
Kingsley & Keith (Chemicals)
  Ltd.
Millwards Merchandise Ltd.
Pfizer Ltd.
Sherman & Co., Ltd.
John & E. Sturge Ltd.

ACID (THIOGLYCOLLIC) and Salts
Victor Blagden & Co., Ltd.
Cyclo Chemicals Ltd.
Dunn Bros. Manchester, Ltd.
Evans Chemicals Ltd.
Robinson Brothers Ltd.
Sherman Chemicals Ltd.

AGAR-AGAR
V. Berg & Sons, Ltd.
Berk Ltd.
Bush Boake Allen Ltd.,
  Perfumery Division
T. M. Duché & Sons (U.K.),
  Ltd.
H. J. Evans & Co., Ltd.
Joseph Flach & Sons, Ltd.
H. Frischmann
The General Chemical Co.,
  Ltd.
Geo. T. Gurr Ltd.
F. Gutkind & Co., Ltd.
Impag (London) Ltd.
John Kellys (London) Ltd.

ALBUMEN
V. Berg & Sons, Ltd.
T. M. Duché & Sons (U.K.)
  Ltd.
H. Frischmann
Geo. T. Gurr Ltd.
John Kellys (London) Ltd.

ALCOHOL (AMYL)
Barter Trading Corporation
  Ltd.
Victor Blagden & Co., Ltd.
Bush Boake Allen Ltd.,
  Perfumery Division
James Burrough Ltd.
Rex Campbell & Co., Ltd.
The General Chemical Co.,
  Ltd.
Kingsley & Keith (Chemicals),
  Ltd.
Pharmachim – Sofia

167

A. Revai & Co. (Chemicals),
Ltd.
Tar Residuals Ltd.

ALCOHOL (BENZYL)
Bush Boake Allen Ltd.,
Perfumery Division
Rex Campbell & Co., Ltd.
May & Baker Ltd.
Standard Synthetics Ltd.

ALCOHOL (BUTYL)
Alcohols Ltd.
Barter Trading Corporation
Ltd.
Rex Campbell & Co., Ltd.
Imperial Chemical Industries
Ltd.
Methylating Co., Ltd.
Sherman Chemicals Ltd.
Tar Residuals Ltd.

ALCOHOLS, CETYL and STEARYL
Bio-Cosmetics Research
Laboratories
Victor Blagden & Co., Ltd.
Rex Campbell & Co., Ltd.
Croda Ltd.
Cyclo Chemicals Ltd.
Givaudan & Co., Ltd
Glovers (Chemicals) Ltd.
Keegan Dyestuffs &
Chemicals Ltd.
Kingsley & Keith (Chemicals)
Ltd.
Marchon Products Ltd.
Price's (Bromborough) Ltd.
Ronsheim & Moore Ltd.

ALCOHOL (ETHYL)
See under **Alcohols
(I.M.S.)** *and* **(S.V.R.)**

ALCOHOLS, FATTY
Victor Blagden & Co., Ltd.
Croda Ltd.
Cyclo Chemicals Ltd.
Givaudan & Co., Ltd.
Glovers (Chemicals) Ltd.
Keegan Dyestuffs &
Chemicals Ltd.
E. J. R. Lovelock
Marchon Products Ltd.
L. R. B. Pearce Ltd.
Price's (Bromborough), Ltd.
Ronsheim & Moore Ltd.

ALCOHOL (I.M.S.)
Alcohols Ltd.

Barter Trading Corporation
Ltd.
Distillers Co., Ltd.
The General Chemical Co.,
Ltd.
May & Baker Ltd.
Methylating Co., Ltd.

ALCOHOL (ISOBUTYL)
Barter Trading Corporation
Ltd.
The General Chemical Co.,
Ltd.
Imperial Chemical Industries
Ltd.
Kingsley & Keith (Chemicals)
Ltd.
Sherman Chemicals Ltd.

ALCOHOL (ISOPROPYL)
Alcohols Ltd.
Barter Trading Corporation
Ltd.
British Celanese Ltd.
James Burrough Ltd.
The General Chemical Co.,
Ltd.
Honeywill & Stein Ltd.
Howards of Ilford Ltd.
Imperial Chemical Industries
Ltd.
Methylating Co., Ltd.
Millwards Merchandise Ltd.
A. Revai & Co. (Chemicals),
Ltd.
Shell Chemical U.K. Ltd.
Standard Synthetics Ltd.

ALCOHOL (METHYL)
Alcohols Ltd.
Barter Trading Corporation
Ltd.
James Burrough Ltd.
The General Chemical Co.,
Ltd.
Imperial Chemical Industries
Ltd.
The Methylating Co., Ltd.
J. M. Steel & Co., Ltd.
Tar Residuals Ltd.

ALCOHOL (OLEYL)
Victor Blagden & Co., Ltd.
Croda Ltd.
Cyclo Chemicals Ltd.
Glovers (Chemicals) Ltd.
Keegan Dyestuffs &
Chemicals Ltd.
Price's (Bromborough) Ltd.

Wynmouth Lehr & Fatoils
Ltd.

ALCOHOL (POLYVINYL)
See under **Polyvinyl
compounds**

ALCOHOL (S.V.R.)
Alcohols Ltd.
James Burrough Ltd.
The General Chemical Co.,
Ltd.
Methylating Co., Ltd.

ALCOHOLS (SULPHONATED FATTY)
Continental Chemical Co.
Cyclo Chemicals Ltd.
Norman Evans & Rais Ltd.
Glovers (Chemicals) Ltd.
Guest Industrials Ltd.
Imperial Chemical Industries
Ltd.
Keegan Dyestuffs &
Chemicals Ltd.
Lankro Chemicals Ltd.
Ronsheim & Moore Ltd.
Sipon Products Ltd.
Sylbeem Laboratories Ltd.

ALKALI-RESISTING WARE
Hathernware Ltd.
Prodorite Ltd.

ALKALIS (GENERAL)
Alcock (Peroxide) Ltd.
British Hydrological
Corporation
Gerard-Polysulphin Ltd.
Sherman Chemicals Ltd.

ALKYLOLAMIDES, FATTY ACID
Continental Chemical Co.
Cyclo Chemicals Ltd.
Dutton & Reinisch Ltd.
Glovers (Chemicals) Ltd.
Keegan Dyestuffs &
Chemicals Ltd.
Lankro Chemicals Ltd.
E. J. R. Lovelock
Price's (Bromborough) Ltd.

ALLANTOIN & ALLANTOINATES
BASF United Kingdom Ltd.
Victor Blagden & Co., Ltd.
Kingsley & Keith (Chemicals)
Ltd.

Chas. Zimmermann & Co.,
Ltd.

ALUM
Jessop & Co.
Laporte Industries Ltd.
(General Chemicals
Division–Widnes)
Shearman & Co., Ltd.
Peter Spence & Sons, Ltd.
Thew Arnott & Co., Ltd.

ALUMINIUM (METALLIC POWDER)
BASF United Kingdom Ltd.
Berk Ltd.
Blackwell's Metallurgical
Works Ltd.

ALUMINIUM CHLORHYDRATE
Albright & Wilson (Mfg.)
Ltd.
Hoechst Chemicals Ltd.
Sherman Chemicals Ltd.
Wilfrid Smith (Fine
Chemicals) Ltd.

ALUMINIUM CHLORIDE
BASF United Kingdom Ltd.
Berk Ltd.
The General Chemical Co.,
Ltd.
Imperial Chemical Industries
Ltd.
Kingsley & Keith (Chemicals)
Ltd.
Peter Spence & Sons, Ltd.
Tar Residuals Ltd.

ALUMINIUM HYDROXIDE
Bush Beach & Segner Bayley
Ltd.
Laporte Industries Ltd.
(General Chemicals
Division–Widnes)
Thomas Morson & Son, Ltd.
C. E. Ramsden & Co., Ltd.
Wilfrid Smith (Fine
Chemicals) Ltd.
Stanley G. Walker & Co.,
Ltd.

ALUMINIUM OXIDE
Bush Beach & Segner Bayley
Ltd.
Kingsley & Keith (Chemicals)
Ltd.

C. E. Ramsden & Co., Ltd.
Tar Residuals Ltd.

ALUMINIUM SILICATE
Bush Beach & Segner Bayley
Ltd.
Joseph Crosfield & Sons, Ltd.
Durham Raw Materials Ltd.
Hardman & Holden Ltd.

ALUMINIUM STEARATE
A.B.M. Industrial Products
Ltd.
Bush Boake Allen Ltd.,
Perfumery Division
Durham Raw Materials Ltd.
Norman Evans & Rais Ltd.
Hardman & Holden Ltd.
Imperial Chemical Industries
Ltd.
Wilfrid Smith (Fine
Chemicals Ltd.
Peter Spence & Sons, Ltd.
Stanley G. Walker & Co.,
Ltd.

ALUMINIUM SULPHATE
H. J. Evans & Co., Ltd.
The General Chemical Co.,
Ltd.
Jessop & Co.
Laporte Industries Ltd.
(General Chemicals
Division–Widnes)
Sherman Chemicals Ltd.

AMBERGRIS, AMBER RESIN
Bertrand Freres Ltd.
Charabot & Cie Ltd.
H. E. Daniel Ltd.
Dragoco (Gt. Britain) Ltd.
Dubuis & Rowsell Ltd.
Fuerst Day Lawson Ltd.
A. J. Gomiero Ltd. (V. Mane
Fils S.A.)
Lockwood, Magrath Pty.,
Ltd.
McVittie, Anderson & Co.,
Ltd.
A. W. Munns & Co., Ltd.
Roure Bertrand Fils et Justin
Dupont
P. Samuelson & Co., Ltd.
R. Sarant & Co., Ltd.
R. C. Treatt & Co., Ltd.
Alfred Paul White & Son

AMIDES, FATTY
Armour Hess Chemicals Ltd.
Victor Blagden & Co., Ltd.
Cyclo Chemicals Ltd.
Dutton & Reinisch Ltd.
Glovers (Chemicals) Ltd.
Guest Industrials Ltd.
Honeywill & Stein Ltd.
Keegan Dyestuff & Chemicals
Ltd.
Lankro Chemicals Ltd.
E. J. R. Lovelock
Price's (Bromborough) Ltd.
J. C. Thompson & Co.
(Duron), Ltd.
Shell Chemical U.K. Ltd.

AMINES, ALIPHATIC
Armour Hess Chemicals Ltd.
Victor Blagden & Co., Ltd.
British Hydrological
Corporation
Glovers (Chemicals) Ltd.

AMINES, FATTY
Armour Hess Chemicals Ltd.
Cyclo Chemicals Ltd.
Glovers (Chemicals) Ltd.
Guest Industrials Ltd.
Hoechst Chemicals Ltd.
Marchon Products Ltd.

AMMONIA
Associated Chemical
Companies (Mfg.) Ltd.
Barter Trading Corporation
Ltd.
Berk Ltd.
The General Chemical Co.,
Ltd.
Imperial Chemical Industries
Ltd.
Laporte Industries Ltd.
(General Chemicals
Division–Leeds)
London Tar & Chemical Co.,
Ltd.
May & Baker Ltd.
Millwards Merchandize Ltd.
Scottish Tar Distillers Ltd.
Sherman Chemicals Ltd.

AMMONIUM ACETATE
A.B.M. Industrial Products
Ltd.
Frederick Allen & Sons
(Chemicals), Ltd.
Berk Ltd.

The General Chemical Co.,
Ltd.
Millwards Merchandise Ltd.
Sherman Chemicals Ltd.
Tar Residuals Ltd.

AMMONIUM
BICARBONATE
Associated Chemical
Companies (Mfg.) Ltd.
BASF United Kingdom Ltd.
The General Chemical Co.,
Ltd.
Jessop & Co.
Thomas Morson & Son, Ltd.
Tar Residuals Ltd.

AMMONIUM
CARBONATE
Associated Chemical
Companies (Mfg.) Ltd.
BASF United Kingdom Ltd.
The General Chemical Co.,
Ltd.
Jessop & Co.
Thomas Morson & Son, Ltd.
Tar Residuals Ltd.

AMMONIUM CHLORIDE
A.B.M. Industrial Products
Ltd.
BASF United Kingdom Ltd.
Berk Ltd.
H. J. Evans & Co., Ltd.
The General Chemical Co.,
Ltd.
Howards of Ilford Ltd.
Imperial Chemical Industries
Ltd.
Laporte Industries Ltd.
(Organics & Pigments
Division–Ilford)
Millwards Merchandise Ltd.
Thomas Morson & Son, Ltd.
Sherman Chemicals Ltd.
Tar Residuals Ltd.

AMMONIUM SULPHIDE
SOLUTION
Frederick Allen & Sons
(Chemicals), Ltd.

AMMONIUM SULPHITE
A.B.M. Industrial Products
Ltd.
Sherman Chemicals Ltd.

AMMONIUM
THIOGLYCOLLATE
Cyclo Chemicals Ltd.

Dunn Bros. Manchester Ltd.
Evans Chemicals Ltd.
Robinson Brothers Ltd.

AMPHOLYTES
Cyclo Chemicals Ltd.
Dutton & Reinisch Ltd.
Glovers (Chemicals) Ltd.
Guest Industrials Ltd.
Ronsheim & Moore Ltd.

AMPHOTERIC S.A.
AGENTS
Alwitt Ltd.
Cyclo Chemicals Ltd.
Dutton & Reinisch Ltd.
Fine Dyestuffs & Chemicals
Ltd.
Glovers (Chemicals) Ltd.
Guest Industrials Ltd.
Lennig Chemicals Ltd.
Ronsheim & Moore Ltd.

AMYL ACETATE
Victor Blagden & Co., Ltd.
Bush Boake Allen Ltd.,
Perfumery Division
Rex Campbell & Co., Ltd.
Cyclo Chemicals Ltd.
The General Chemical Co.,
Ltd.
Standard Synthetics Ltd.
Tar Residuals Ltd.
White Tomkins & Courage
Ltd.

AMYL BUTYRATE
Bush Boake Allen Ltd.,
Perfumery Division
Food Industries Ltd.
Standard Synthetics Ltd.

ANGELICA OILS
Bertrand Freres Ltd.
Bush Boake Allen Ltd.,
Perfumery Division
Charabot & Cie Ltd.
H. E. Daniel Ltd.
Dragoco (Gt. Britain) Ltd.
Food Industries Ltd.
Gale & Mount Ltd.
A. J. Gomiero Ltd. (V. Mane
Fils S.A.)
Lautier Fils Ltd.
A. W. Munns & Co., Ltd.
'Naarden' (London) Ltd.
Natural & Synthetic
Perfumery Essence Co.

Roure Bertrand Fils et Justin
Dupont
H. E. Stringer Ltd.
R. C. Treatt & Co., Ltd.
Alfred Paul White & Son
White, Tomkins & Courage
Ltd.
Wilson & Mansfield Ltd.
Chas. Zimmermann & Co.,
Ltd.

ANISEED OIL
V. Berg & Sons, Ltd.
Bertrand Freres Ltd.
Blyth, Greene, Jourdain &
Co., Ltd.
Bruce, Starke & Co., Ltd.
Bush Boake Allen Ltd.,
Perfumery Division
Charabot & Cie Ltd.
F. D. Copeland & Sons Ltd.
Courtin & Warner Ltd.
H. E. Daniel Ltd.
Felton Co. (Gt. Britain) Ltd.
Food Industries Ltd.
Fuerst Day Lawson Ltd.
Gale & Mount Ltd.
A. J. Gomiero Ltd. (V. Mane
Fils S.A.)
T. Harrison & Co., Ltd.
A. G. Hersom
W. H. Hobbs & Co., Ltd.
Hollander Hyams Ltd.
Hollands Distillery (Essential
Oils) Ltd.
John Kellys (London) Ltd.
Lautier Fils Ltd.
A. W. Munns & Co., Ltd.
Pigalle (International) Ltd.
Roure Bertrand Fils et Justin
Dupont
R. Sarant & Co., Ltd.
Standard Synthetics Ltd.
Tar Residuals Ltd.
R. C. Treatt & Co., Ltd.
Alfred Paul White & Son
White, Tomkins & Courage
Ltd.
Wilson & Mansfield Ltd.
Chas. Zimmermann & Co., Ltd.

ANNATTO
D. F. Anstead Ltd.
V. Berg & Sons, Ltd.
Blyth, Greene, Jourdain &
Co., Ltd.
Joseph Flach & Sons, Ltd.

170

Food Industries Ltd.
H. Frischmann
F. Gutkind & Co., Ltd.
John Kellys (London) Ltd.
Pfizer Ltd.

ANTIOXIDANTS
See also **Preservatives**
Berk Ltd.
Bush Boake Allen Ltd.,
    Perfumery Division
Coalite & Chemical Products
    Ltd.
Dragoco (Gt. Britain) Ltd.
Glovers (Chemicals) Ltd.
Guest Industrials Ltd.
Honeywill & Stein Ltd.
Imperial Chemical Industries
    Ltd.
Kingsley & Keith (Chemicals)
    Ltd.
Laporte Industries Ltd.
    (Organics & Pigments
    Division–Ilford)
May & Baker Ltd.
'Naarden' (London) Ltd.
Nipa Laboratories Ltd.
A. Revai & Co. (Chemicals)
    Ltd.
Roche Products Ltd.
Shell Chemical U.K. Ltd.
Sherman Chemicals Ltd.
Ward, Blenkinsop & Co., Ltd.

AROMATIC CHEMICALS (SYNTHETICS AND ISOLATES)
Aromatica Ltd.
Bertrand Freres Ltd.
Birmingham Chemical Co.,
    Ltd.
Victor Blagden & Co., Ltd.
Bruce, Starke & Co., Ltd.
Bush Boake Allen Ltd.,
    Perfumery Division
Rex Campbell & Co., Ltd.
Charabot & Cie Ltd.
Ciba Clayton Ltd.
Cocker Chemical Co. Ltd.
H. E. Daniel Ltd.
Dragoco (Gt. Britain) Ltd.
Esrolko Ltd.
Field & Co. (Aromatics), Ltd.
Firmenich Ltd.
Food Industries Ltd.
Gale & Mount Ltd.
Givaudan & Co., Ltd.
Haarman & Reimer Ltd.

T. Harrison & Co., Ltd.
Hoechst Chemicals Ltd.
International Flavours &
    Fragrances I.F.F. (Gt.
    Britain) Ltd.
Kingsley & Keith (Chemicals)
    Ltd.
H. M. Langton & Co., Ltd.
Lockwood, Magrath Pty.,
    Ltd.
May & Baker Ltd.
A. W. Munns & Co., Ltd.
'Naarden' (London) Ltd.
Natural & Synthetic
    Perfumery Essence Co.
Nipa Laboratories Ltd.
Norda-Schimmel
    International Ltd.
P. T. Petley & Co., Ltd.
Proprietary Perfumes Ltd.
Roche Products Ltd.
Roure Bertrand Fils et Justin
    Dupont
P. Samuelson & Co. Ltd.
R. Sarant & Co., Ltd.
Söflor Ltd.
Standard Synthetics Ltd.
Staveley Chemicals Ltd.
H. E. Stringer Ltd.
Tar Residuals Ltd.
Alfred Paul White & Son
Wilson & Mansfield Ltd.
*See also the list of suppliers
given under* **Perfumery
compounds** *and other specific
headings.*

BARIUM SULPHIDE
Sherman Chemicals Ltd.

BASIL
Bertrand Freres Ltd.
Charabot & Cie Ltd.
F. D. Copeland & Sons, Ltd.
Food Industries Ltd.
Fuerst Day Lawson Ltd.
Gale & Mount Ltd.
A. J. Gomiero Ltd. (V. Mane
    Fils S.A.)
A. W. Munns & Co., Ltd.
Roure Bertrand Fils et Justin
    Dupont
R. Sarant & Co., Ltd.
H. E. Stringer Ltd.
Alfred Paul White & Son
Wilson & Mansfield Ltd.

BAY
Blyth, Greene, Jourdain &
    Co., Ltd.
Bruce, Starke & Co., Ltd.
Buch Boake Allen Ltd.,
    Perfumery Division
H. E. Daniel Ltd.
Food Industries Ltd.
Lautier Fils Ltd.
Fuerst Day Lawson Ltd.
Gale & Mount Ltd.
W. H. Hobbs & Co., Ltd.
A. W. Munns & Co., Ltd.
Roure Bertrand Fils et Justin
    Dupont
R. Sarant & Co., Ltd.
R. C. Treatt & Co., Ltd.
Chas. Zimmermann & Co., Ltd

BENTONITE
D. F. Anstead Ltd.
Berk Ltd.
Bush Beach & Segner Bayley
    Ltd.
H. J. Evans & Co., Ltd.
Fullers Earth Union Ltd.
Laporte Industries Ltd.
    (Organics and pigments
    Division–Redhill)
Colin Stewart Ltd.

BENZOYL PEROXIDE
Imperial Chemical Industries
    Ltd.
Kingsley & Keith (Chemicals)
    Ltd.
Laporte Industries Ltd.
    (General Chemicals
    Division–Luton)
Novadel Ltd.

BERGAMOT OIL
Bertrand Freres Ltd.
Blyth, Greene, Jourdain & Co.,
    Ltd.
Bush Boake Allen Ltd.,
    Perfumery Division
Charabot & Cie Ltd.
Antoine Chiris Ltd.
H. E. Daniel Ltd.
Dragoco (Gt. Britain) Ltd.
Dubuis & Rowsell Ltd.
Food Industries Ltd.
Fuerst Day Lawson Ltd.
Gale & Mount Ltd.
A. J. Gomiero Ltd. (V. Mane
    Fils S.A.)
Geo. T. Gurr Ltd.
F. Gutkind & Co., Ltd.

A. G. Hersom
W. H. Hobbs & Co., Ltd.
H. M. Langton & Co., Ltd.
Lautier Fils Ltd.
Mallagh & Co.
A. W. Munns & Co., Ltd.
Natural & Synthetic
Perfumery Essence Co.
Norda-Schimmel International
Ltd.
Pigalle (International) Ltd.
William Ransom & Son, Ltd.
Roure Bertrand Fils et Justin
Dupont
P. Samuelson & Co., Ltd.
R. Sarant & Co., Ltd.
Sōflor Ltd.
Standard Synthetics Ltd.
R. C. Treatt & Co., Ltd.
Alfred Paul White & Son
Wilson & Mansfield Ltd.
Chas. Zimmermann & Co.,
Ltd.

BETA-METHYL
UMBELLIFERONE
The General Chemical Co.,
Ltd.
Honeywill & Stein Ltd.
Kingsley & Keith (Chemicals)
Ltd.

BETA NAPHTHOL
BASF United Kingdom Ltd.
Victor Blagden & Co., Ltd.
Geo. T. Gurr Ltd.
Imperial Chemical Industries
Ltd.
Kingsley & Keith (Chemicals)
Ltd.
Millwards Merchandise Ltd.
Tar Residuals Ltd.

BLACKS (CARBON)
D. F. Anstead Ltd.
Blackwell's Metallurgical
Works Ltd.
Bush Beach and Segner Bayley
Ltd.
Butterfield Laboratories Ltd.
Ciba Clayton Ltd.
R. W. Greeff & Co., Ltd.
Stanley G. Walker & Co., Ltd.
Williams (Hounslow) Ltd.

BLACKS (LAMP,
VEGETABLE)
D. F. Anstead Ltd.

Bush Beach & Segner Bayley
Ltd.
W. Hawley & Son, Ltd.
Procter Johnson & Co., Ltd.
Shearman & Co., Ltd.

BLANC FIXE
Berk Ltd.
H. J. Evans & Co., Ltd.
Imperial Smelting Corporation
(Sales) Ltd.
J. M. Steel & Co., Ltd.
Stanley G. Walker & Co. Ltd.

BOIS DE ROSE OIL
V. Berg & Sons, Ltd.
Blyth, Greene, Jourdain & Co.,
Ltd.
Bush Boake Allen Ltd.,
Perfumery Division
Charabot & Cie Ltd.
Antoine Chiris Ltd.
F. D. Copeland & Sons, Ltd.
H. E. Daniel Ltd.
Felton Co. (Gt. Britain), Ltd.
Food Industries Ltd.
Fuerst Day Lawson Ltd.
Gale & Mount Ltd.
A. J. Gomiero Ltd. (V. Mane
Fils S.A.)
W. H. Hobbs & Co., Ltd.
Hollander Hyams Ltd.
Lautier Fils Ltd.
A. W. Munns & Co. Ltd.
Roure Bertrand Fils et Justin
Dupont
R. Sarant & Co., Ltd.
R. C. Treatt & Co., Ltd.
White Tomkins & Courage
Ltd.
Wilson & Mansfield Ltd.
Chas. Zimmermann & Co.,
Ltd.

BORAX
Borax & Chemicals Ltd.
Borax Consolidated Ltd.
Durham Raw Materials Ltd.
H. J. Evans & Co., Ltd.
Geo. T. Gurr Ltd.
Thomas Morson & Son, Ltd.
Patent Borax Co., Ltd.
Geo. H. Poole & Son (Bootle),
Ltd.
Harry B. Wood Ltd.

BRILLIANTINE OILS
See **Oils, mineral**

BROMO ACID
See under **Colours** and
Dyestuffs

BROMSTYROLE
Bush Boake Allen Ltd.,
Perfumery Division
Gale & Mount Ltd.
Givaudan & Co., Ltd.
A. W. Munns & Co., Ltd.

BUTYL ACETATE
Barter Trading Corporation
Ltd.
Rex Campbell & Co., Ltd.
The General Chemical Co.,
Ltd.
Methylating Co., Ltd.
Tar Residuals Ltd.

BUTYL LACTATE
Rex Campbell & Co., Ltd.

CALAMINE
Durham Raw Materials Ltd.
Howards of Ilford Ltd.
H. Lattimer
Thomas Morson & Son, Ltd.
Sherman Chemicals Ltd.

CALCINED MAGNESIA
See **Magnesium oxide**

CALCIUM CARBONATE
PRECIPITATED
Richard Baker & Co., Ltd.
Victor Blagden & Co., Ltd.
Blackwell's Metallurgical
Works Ltd.
Chalk Products Ltd.
Dunn Bros. Manchester Ltd.
H. J. Evans & Co., Ltd.
A Levermore & Co., Ltd.
Thomas Morson & Son, Ltd.
L. R. B. Pearce Ltd.
Scott Bader & Co., Ltd.
Shearman & Co., Ltd.
John & E. Sturge Ltd.
Thew Arnott & Co., Ltd.

CALCIUM CHLORIDE
A. Elder Reed & Co., Ltd.
The General Chemical Co.,
Ltd.
Howards of Ilford Ltd.
Imperial Chemical Industries
Ltd.
Millwards Merchandise Ltd.
L. R. B. Pearce Ltd.
Sherman Chemicals Ltd.

Tar Residuals Ltd.

CALCIUM HYDROXIDE
The General Chemical Co., Ltd.
Imperial Chemical Industries Ltd.

CALCIUM PHOSPHATES
Thomas Morson & Son, Ltd.
L. R. B. Pearce Ltd.

CALCIUM PROPIONATE
Distillers Chemicals & Plastics Ltd.

CALCIUM SILICATE
Blackwell's Metallurgical Works Ltd.
Joseph Crosfield & Sons, Ltd.
Durham Raw Materials Ltd.
Johns-Manville (Gt. Britain) Ltd.

CALGON
See **Sodium Hexametaphosphate**

CAMPHOR
V. Berg & Sons, Ltd.
Blyth, Greene, Jourdain & Co., Ltd.
Courtin & Warner Ltd.
H. E. Daniel Ltd.
H. Frischmann
Fuerst Day Lawson Ltd.
Howards of Ilford Ltd.
Langley-Smith & Co., Ltd.
Laporte Industries Ltd.
(Organics & Pigments Division–Ilford)
R. Sarant & Co., Ltd.
Standard Synthetics Ltd.
Techno Chemical Industries Ltd.
R. C. Treatt & Co. Ltd.
A. & M. Zimmermann
Chas. Zimmermann & Co., Ltd.

CAMPHOR OIL
V. Berg & Sons, Ltd.
Blyth, Greene, Jourdain & Co., Ltd.
Bush Boake Allen Ltd., Perfumery Division
Charabot & Cie Ltd.
Courtin & Warner Ltd.
H. E. Daniel Ltd.
Food Industries Ltd.
Fuerst Day Lawson Ltd

Gale & Mount Ltd.
W. H. Hobbs & Co., Ltd.
Roure Bertrand Fils et Justin Dupont
R. Sarant & Co., Ltd.
Standard Synthetics Ltd.
Techno Chemical Industries Ltd.
R. C. Treatt & Co., Ltd.
Wilson & Mansfield Ltd.
Chas. Zimmermann & Co., Ltd.

CANANGA OIL
V. Berg & Sons, Ltd.
Blyth, Greene, Jourdain & Co., Ltd.
Bush Boake Allen Ltd., Perfumery Division
Charabot & Cie Ltd.
Antoine Chiris Ltd.
F. D. Copeland & Sons, Ltd.
H. E. Daniel Ltd.
Fuerst Day Lawson Ltd.
Gale & Mount Ltd.
A. J. Gomiero Ltd. (V. Mane Fils S.A.)
F. Gutkind & Co., Ltd.
A. G. Hersom
Lautier Fils Ltd.
Mallagh & Co.
A. W. Munns & Co., Ltd.
Roure Bertrand Fils et Justin Dupont
R. Sarant & Co., Ltd.
Standard Synthetics Ltd.
R. C. Treatt & Co., Ltd.
Alfred Paul White & Son
Wilson & Mansfield Ltd.
Chas. Zimmermann & Co., Ltd.

CARAWAY OIL
Bush Boake Allen Ltd., Perfumery Division
Charabot & Cie Ltd.
Courtin & Warner Ltd.
H. E. Daniel Ltd.
Dragoco (Gt. Britain) Ltd.
Food Industries Ltd.
Fuerst Day Lawson Ltd.
Gale & Mount Ltd.
W. H. Hobbs & Co., Ltd.
Hollands Distillery (Essential Oils) Ltd.
Lautier Fils Ltd.
J. & G. Miller
A. W. Munns & Co., Ltd.

'Naarden' (London) Ltd.
Roure Bertrand Fils et Justin Dupont
Standard Synthetics Ltd.
Alfred Paul White & Son
White, Tomkins & Courage Ltd.
Wilson & Mansfield Ltd.
Chas. Zimmermann & Co., Ltd.

CARBITOL
See **Diethylene glycol monoethyl ether**

CARBOLIC ACID
See under **Phenol**

CARBON TETRACHLORIDE
Honeywill & Stein Ltd.
Kingsley & Keith (Chemicals) Ltd.
May & Baker Ltd.
Thomas Morson & Son, Ltd.
Sherman Chemicals Ltd.

CARBOXYL METHYL CELLULOSE
Berk Ltd.
Victor Blagden & Co., Ltd.
British Celanese Ltd.
Courtaulds Ltd.
Fine Dyestuffs & Chemicals Ltd.
The General Chemical Co., Ltd.
Hercules Powder Co., Ltd.
Hoechst Chemicals Ltd.
Honeywill & Stein Ltd.
Imperial Chemical Industries Ltd.
Price's (Bromborough) Ltd.
Union Carbide Ltd. (Chemical Division)

CARMINE
D. F. Anstead Ltd.
Butterfield Laboratories Ltd.
Courtin & Warner Ltd.
Food Industries Ltd.
A. J. Gomiero Ltd. (V. Mane Fils S.A.)
F. Gutkind & Co., Ltd.
R. Sarant & Co., Ltd.
Roure Bertrand Fils et Justin Dupont
Stanley G. Walker & Co., Ltd.
Chas. Zimmermann & Co., Ltd.

CAROTENE
D. F. Anstead Ltd.
Food Industries Ltd.
Wm. Ransom & Son, Ltd.
Roche Products Ltd.

CARRAGHEEN MOSS
J. W. Cumming and Son, Ltd.
T. M. Duché & Sons (U.K.),
Ltd.
Joseph Flach & Sons, Ltd.
H. Frischmann
M. Hamburger & Sons, Ltd.
A. Revai & Co. (Chemicals),
Ltd.

CARROT SEED OIL
Bertrand Freres Ltd.
Bio-Cosmetic Research
Laboratories
Charabot & Cie Ltd.
Antoine Chiris Ltd.
H. E. Daniel Ltd.
Dragoco (Gt. Britain) Ltd.
Food Industries Ltd.
Gale & Mount Ltd.
A. J. Gomiero Ltd. (V. Mane
Fils S.A.)
Lautier Fils Ltd.
A. W. Munns & Co., Ltd.
Natural & Synthetic Perfumery
Essence Co.
Roure Bertrand Fils et Justin
Dupont
R. Sarant & Co., Ltd.
H. E. Stringer Ltd.
Alfred Paul White & Son

**CARVONES (LAEVO-
and DEXTRO-)**
H. E. Daniel Ltd.
Dragoco (Gt. Britain) Ltd.
Gale & Mount Ltd.

CASCARILLA OIL
Bush Boake Allen Ltd.,
Perfumery Division
H. E. Daniel Ltd.
Joseph Flach & Sons, Ltd.
H. Frischmann
William Ransom & Son, Ltd.
R. Sarant & Co., Ltd.
R. C. Treatt & Co., Ltd.
Wilson & Mansfield Ltd.

CASEIN
Casein (Industries) Ltd.
Hiron & Rempler Ltd.

Kingsley & Keith (Chemicals)
Ltd.
Harry B. Wood Ltd.
Wynmouth Lehr & Fatoils Ltd.

CASSIA OIL
V. Berg & Sons, Ltd.
Bertrand Freres Ltd.
Blyth, Greene, Jourdain & Co.,
Ltd.
Bush Boake Allen Ltd.,
Perfumery Division
Charabot & Cie Ltd.
H. E. Daniel Ltd.
Dragoco (Gt. Britain) Ltd.
Dubuis & Rowsell Ltd.
Food Industries Ltd.
Fuerst Day Lawson Ltd.
Gale & Mount Ltd.
W. H. Hobbs & Co., Ltd.
John Kellys (London) Ltd.
R. Sarant & Co., Ltd.
Sõflor Ltd.
Standard Synthetics Ltd.
R. C. Treatt & Co., Ltd.
Wilson & Mansfield Ltd.
Chas. Zimmermann & Co.,
Ltd.

CASTOREUM
Bertrand Freres Ltd.
Charabot & Cie Ltd.
Antoine Chiris Ltd.
H. E. Daniel Ltd.
Fuerst Day Lawson Ltd.
Lautier Fils Ltd.
A. W. Munns & Co., Ltd.
P. Samuelson & Co., Ltd.
H. E. Stringer Ltd.
R. C. Treatt & Co., Ltd.
Alfred Paul White & Son
Wilson & Mansfield Ltd.

CATIONIC S.A. AGENTS
Alwitt Ltd.
Victor Blagden & Co., Ltd.
Rex Campbell & Co., Ltd.
Ciba Clayton Ltd.
Cyclo Chemicals Ltd.
Dutton & Reinisch Ltd.
Fine Dyestuffs & Chemicals
Ltd.
Glovers (Chemicals) Ltd.
Hoechst Chemicals Ltd.
Keegan Dyestuffs & Chemicals
Ltd.
Marchon Products Ltd.
Ronsheim & Moore Ltd.

**CAUSTIC POTASH &
CAUSTIC SODA**
See **Potassium hydroxide**
and **Sodium hydroxide**

CEDARWOOD OIL
V. Berg & Sons, Ltd.
Bertrand Freres Ltd.
Blyth, Greene, Jourdain & Co.,
Ltd.
Bruce, Starke & Co., Ltd.
Bush Boake Allen Ltd.,
Perfumery Division
Charabot & Cie Ltd.
F. D. Copeland & Sons, Ltd.
Courtin & Warner Ltd.
H. E. Daniel Ltd.
Dragoco (Gt. Britain) Ltd.
Felton Company (Great
Britain) Ltd.
Fuerst Day Lawson Ltd.
Gale & Mount Ltd.
A. J. Gomiero Ltd. (V. Mane
Fils S.A.)
Geo. T. Gurr Ltd.
F. Gutkind & Co., Ltd.
A. G. Hersom
W. H. Hobbs & Co., Ltd.
Hollander Hyams Ltd.
Imperial Chemical Industries
Ltd.
Lautier Fils Ltd.
A. W. Munns & Co., Ltd.
Norda-Schimmel International
Ltd.
Roure Bertrand Fils et Justin
Dupont
P. Samuelson & Co., Ltd.
R. Sarant & Co., Ltd.
Standard Synthetics Ltd.
R. C. Treatt & Co., Ltd.
Wilson & Mansfield Ltd.
Chas. Zimmermann & Co.,
Ltd.

**CHALK (PREPARED
AND PRECIPITATED)**
Blackwell's Metallurgical
Works Ltd.
Harry B. Wood Ltd.
A. & M. Zimmermann

CHALK (FRENCH)
See under **Talc**

CHARCOAL (ANIMAL)
Harrison, Clark Ltd.
Shearman & Co., Ltd.

CHARCOAL (WOOD)
Bush Beach & Segner Bayley Ltd.
R. W. Greeff & Co., Ltd.
Harrison, Clark Ltd.
Shearman & Co., Ltd.
Roche Products Ltd.
Shearman & Co., Ltd.
Sherman Chemicals Ltd.
John & E. Sturge Ltd.
Ward, Blenkinsop & Co., Ltd.
Chas. Zimmermann & Co., Ltd.

CHINA CLAY
Richard Baker & Co., Ltd.
Berk Ltd.
Durham Raw Materials Ltd.
English Clays Lovering Pochin & Co., Ltd.
H. J. Evans & Co., Ltd.
Kingsley & Keith (Chemicals) Ltd.
H. Lattimer
A. Levermore & Co., Ltd.
Thomas Morson & Son, Ltd.
New Consolidated Mines of Cornwall Ltd.
C. E. Ramsden & Co., Ltd.
Scott Bader & Co., Ltd.
Shearman & Co., Ltd.
Zach Cartwright Ltd.

CHLOROPHYLL
Bio-Cosmetic Research Laboratories
Fredk. Boehm Ltd.
Bush Boake Allen Ltd., Perfumery Division
Food Industries Ltd.
Wm. Ransom & Son, Ltd.

CHOLESTEROL (CHOLESTERIN)
Bio-Cosmetic Research Laboratories

CINNAMON OIL
V. Berg & Sons, Ltd.
Blyth, Greene, Jourdain & Co., Ltd.
Bruce, Starke & Co., Ltd.
Charabot & Cie Ltd.
Courtin & Warner Ltd.
H. E. Daniel Ltd.
Dragoco (Gt. Britain) Ltd.
Felton Co. (Gt. Britain), Ltd.
Food Industries Ltd.

H. Frischmann
Fuerst Day Lawson Ltd.
Gale & Mount Ltd.
A. J. Gomiero Ltd. (V. Mane Fils S.A.)
W. H. Hobbs & Co., Ltd.
Hollander Hyams Ltd.
Lautier Fils Ltd.
A. W. Munns & Co., Ltd.
William Ransom & Son, Ltd.
Roure Bertrand Fils et Justin Dupont
R. Sarant & Co., Ltd.
Söflor Ltd.
Standard Synthetics Ltd.
R. C. Treatt & Co., Ltd.
White, Tomkins & Courage Ltd.
Wilson & Mansfield Ltd.
Chas. Zimmermann & Co., Ltd.

CITRONELLA OILS
V. Berg & Sons, Ltd.
Blyth, Greene, Jourdain & Co., Ltd.
Bush Boake Allen Ltd., Perfumery Division
Charabot & Cie Ltd.
F. D. Copeland & Sons, Ltd.
H. E. Daniel Ltd.
Dragoco (Gt. Britain) Ltd.
Food Industries Ltd.
Fuerst Day Lawson Ltd.
Gale & Mount Ltd.
A. G. Hersom
W. H. Hobbs & Co., Ltd.
Hollander Hyams Ltd.
John Kellys (London) Ltd.
Lautier Fils Ltd.
A. W. Munns & Co., Ltd.
R. Sarant & Co., Ltd.
Standard Synthetics Ltd.
R. C. Treatt & Co., Ltd.
Wilson & Mansfield Ltd.
Chas. Zimmermann & Co., Ltd.

CIVET
Bertrand Freres Ltd.
Charabot & Cie Ltd.
Antoine Chiris Ltd.
H. E. Daniel Ltd.
Dragoco (Gt. Britain) Ltd.
Dubuis & Rowsell Ltd.
Fuerst Day Lawson Ltd.
Gale & Mount Ltd.

A. J. Gomiero Ltd. (V. Mane Fils S.A.)
Lautier Fils Ltd.
A. W. Munns & Co., Ltd.
Roure Bertrand Fils et Justin Dupont
P. Samuelson & Co., Ltd.
R. Sarant & Co., Ltd.
H. E. Stringer Ltd.
R. C. Treatt & Co., Ltd.
Alfred Paul White & Son
Wilson & Mansfield Ltd.

CLOVE OIL
V. Berg & Sons, Ltd.
Bertrand Freres Ltd.
Blyth, Greene, Jourdain & Co., Ltd.
Bush Boake Allen Ltd., Perfumery Division
Charabot & Cie Ltd.
Courtin & Warner Ltd.
H. E. Daniel Ltd.
Dragoco (Gt. Britain) Ltd.
Food Industries Ltd.
H. Frischmann
Gale & Mount Ltd.
A. J. Gomiero Ltd. (V. Mane Fils S.A.)
A. G. Hersom
W. H. Hobbs & Co., Ltd.
John Kellys (London) Ltd.
Lautier Fils Ltd.
A. W. Munns & Co., Ltd.
R. Sarant & Co., Ltd.
Standard Synthetics Ltd.
R. C. Treatt & Co., Ltd.
White, Tomkins & Courage Ltd.
Wilson & Mansfield Ltd.

COAL TAR
See under **Tar products**

COCOA BUTTER
T. M. Duché & Sons (U.K.), Ltd.
H. Lattimer

COCOA BUTTER (DEODORIZED)
H. Lattimer
L. E. Pritchitt & Co., Ltd.

COLLOIDAL CLAYS
See also **China clay**
English Clays Lovering Pochin & Co., Ltd.

COLOURS (for Soaps, Cosmetics, etc.)

See also **Dyestuffs**

D. F. Anstead Ltd.
British Titan Products Co., Ltd.
Bush Boake Allen Ltd., Perfumery Division
Butterfield Laboratories Ltd.
Ciba Clayton Ltd.
Colne Vale Dye & Chemical Co., Ltd.
Dragoco (Gt. Britain) Ltd.
Geigy (U.K.) Ltd.
Golden Valley Colours Ltd.
W. Hawley & Son, Ltd.
Imperial Chemical Industries Ltd.
Pfizer Ltd.
Pronk, Davis & Rusby Ltd.
Reckitts (Colours) Ltd.
Scottish Flavour & Colour Co. Ltd.
Shearman & Co. Ltd.
W. S. Simpson & Co. (The British Aniline Dye & Chemical Works), Ltd.
Stevenson & Howell Ltd.
Stanley G. Walker & Co., Ltd.
Williams (Hounslow) Ltd.

COPPER SULPHATE

Berk Ltd.
British Anhydrous Ammonia Co., Ltd.
H. J. Evans & Co., Ltd.
The General Chemical Co., Ltd.
James Greenshields & Co., Ltd.
Thomas Morson & Son, Ltd.
Sherman Chemicals Ltd.
Tar Residuals Ltd.

CORIANDER OIL

Bertrand Freres Ltd.
Bush Boake Allen Ltd., Perfumery Division
Antoine Chiris Ltd.
F. D. Copeland & Sons, Ltd.
H. E. Daniel Ltd.
Dragoco (Gt. Britain) Ltd.
Food Industries Ltd.
Fuerst Day Lawson Ltd.
Gale & Mount Ltd.
A. J. Gomiero Ltd. (V. Mane Fils S.A.)
W. H. Hobbs & Co., Ltd.
Lautier Fils Ltd.

A. W. Munns & Co., Ltd.
Norda-Schimmel International Ltd.
Roure Bertrand Fils et Justin Dupont
R. Sarant & Co., Ltd.
H. E. Stringer Ltd.
R. C. Treatt & Co., Ltd.
Alfred Paul White & Son
Wilson & Mansfield Ltd.
Chas. Zimmermann & Co., Ltd.

COSTUS OIL

Bertrand Freres Ltd.
Charabot & Cie Ltd.
Antoine Chiris Ltd.
H. E. Daniel Ltd.
Fuerst Day Lawson Ltd.
Gale & Mount Ltd.
A. J. Gomiero Ltd. (V. Mane Fils S.A.)
Lautier Fils Ltd.
A. W. Munns & Co., Ltd.
Natural & Synthetic Perfumery Essence Co.
Roure Bertrand Fils et Justin Dupont
H. E. Stringer Ltd.
Alfred Paul White & Son
Wilson & Mansfield Ltd.

CREOSOTE

James Greenshields & Co., Ltd.
London Tar & Chemical Co., Ltd.
Midland Tar Distillers Ltd.
Thomas Morson & Son, Ltd.
Scottish Tar Distillers Ltd.
Smith & Forrest (Oils) Ltd.
United Coke & Chemical Co., Ltd.
United Steel Companies Ltd.
Westwood MacNeill & Co., Ltd.

DETERGENTS, SPECIAL

Alcock (Peroxide) Ltd.
British Hydrological Corporation
Burmah Oil Trading Ltd.– Lobitos Division
Ciba Clayton Ltd.
Continental Chemical Co.
Co-operative Wholesale society Ltd.
Joseph Crosfield & Sons, Ltd.
Cyclo Chemicals Ltd.

Diversey Ltd.
Dutton & Reinisch Ltd.
Norman Evans & Rais Ltd.
Fine Dyestuffs & Chemicals Ltd.
Food Industries Ltd.
Germstroyd Ltd.
Glovers (Chemicals) Ltd.
Henkel International G.m.b.H.
Hoechst Chemicals Ltd.
Imperial Chemical Industries Ltd.
Jacobson Van Den Berg & Co. (U.K.), Ltd.
Jeyes Group Ltd.
Keegan Dyestuffs & Chemicals Ltd.
Lankro Chemicals Ltd.
Laporte Industries Ltd. (General Chemicals Division–Luton)
L.T.D. Building Products
Marchon Products Ltd.
Patent Borax Co., Ltd.
Pennsalt Ltd. Chemicals Division
Printat Industries Ltd.
Procter & Gamble Ltd.
Ronsheim & Moore Ltd.
Sandeman Bros. Ltd.
Sandoz Products Ltd.
Sherman Chemicals Ltd.
Sipon Products Ltd.
Sylbeem Laboratories Ltd.
Victor Wolf Ltd.

DETERGENTS, SYNTHETIC

Alcock (Peroxide) Ltd.
Bartoline (Hull) Ltd.
Berk Ltd.
Bersel Mfg. Co., Ltd.
British Hydrological Corporation
Ciba Aerochemicals Ltd.
Ciba Clayton Ltd.
Co-operative Wholesale Society Ltd.
Cyclo Chemicals Ltd.
Diversey Ltd.
Dutton & Reinisch Ltd.
Fine Dyestuffs & Chemicals Ltd.
Food Industries Ltd.
Norman Evans & Rais Ltd.
Geigy (U.K.) Ltd.
Germstroyd Ltd.

176

Glovers (Chemicals) Ltd.
Hoechst Chemicals Ltd.
Horton Cleaning Products Ltd.
Hull Chemical Works Ltd.
Imperial Chemical Industries
  Ltd.
Jacobson Van Den Berg & Co.
  (U.K.) Ltd.
Keegan Dyestuffs & Chemicals
  Ltd.
Lankro Chemicals Ltd.
Laporte Industries Ltd.
  (General Chemicals
  Division–Luton)
L.T.D. Building Products
Marchon Products Ltd.
Procter & Gamble Ltd.
Ronsheim & Moore Ltd.
Sandoz Products Ltd.
Shell Chemical U.K. Ltd.
Sipon Products Ltd.
Victor Wolf Ltd.

DIACETIN
See **Glyceryl diacetate**

DIACETYL
Bush Boake Allen Ltd.,
  Perfumery Division
Food Industries Ltd.
Kingsley & Keith (Chemicals)
  Ltd.

DICALCIUM
PHOSPHATE
Guest Industrials Ltd.
Hoechst Chemicals Ltd.
Thomas Morson & Son, Ltd.
L. R. B. Pearce Ltd.

DIETHYL PHTHALATE
Barter Trading Corporation
  Ltd.
Bush Boake Allen Ltd.,
  Perfumery Division

DIETHYLENE GLYCOL
Barter Trading Corporation
  Ltd.
Rex Campbell & Co., Ltd.
The General Chemical Co.,
  Ltd.
R. W. Greeff & Co., Ltd.
Hoechst Chemicals Ltd.
Honeywill & Stein Ltd.
Imperial Chemical Industries
  Ltd.
A. Revai & Co. (Chemicals),
  Ltd.

Shell Chemicals U.K. Ltd.
Union Carbide Ltd.
  (Chemicals Division)

DIETHYLENE GLYCOL
MONOETHYL ETHER
Barter Trading Corporation
  Ltd.
BASF United Kingdom Ltd.
Rex Campbell & Co., Ltd.
The General Chemical Co.,
  Ltd.
R. W. Greeff & Co., Ltd.
Hoechst Chemicals Ltd.
Honeywill & Stein Ltd.
Kingsley & Keith (Chemicals)
  Ltd.
A. Revai & Co. (Chemicals),
  Ltd.
Shell Chemicals U.K. Ltd.
Union Carbide Ltd.
  (Chemicals Division)

DIPENTENE
Bowring, Jones & Tidy Ltd.
H. E. Daniel Ltd.
Hercules Powder Co. Ltd.
Honeywill & Stein Ltd.
Langley-Smith & Co., Ltd.
Meade-King, Robinson & Co.,
  Ltd.
A. V. Pound & Co., Ltd.
Standard Synthetics Ltd.
Tar Residuals Ltd.
White Sea & Baltic Co., P. &
  I. Danischewsky Ltd.
Wynmouth Lehr & Fatoils Ltd.

DISODIUM
PHORYCHATE
See **Sodium phosphate
(Dibasic)**

DYESTUFFS
See also **Colours for soaps,
Cosmetics,** etc.
D. F. Anstead Ltd.
Butterfield Laboratories Ltd.
Ciba Clayton Ltd.
Colne Vale Dye & Chemical
  Co., Ltd.
Dragoco (Gt. Britain) Ltd.
Fine Dyestuffs & Chemicals
  Ltd.
Geigy (U.K.) Ltd.
Geo. T. Gurr Ltd.
Imperial Chemical Industries
  Ltd.
Pronk, Davis & Busby Ltd.

Sandoz Products Ltd.
Shearman & Co. Ltd.
W. S. Simpson & Co. (The
  British Aniline Dye &
  Chemical Works), Ltd.
Stanley G. Walker & Co., Ltd.
Williams (Hounslow) Ltd.
A. & M. Zimmermann

EMERY BOARDS
See **Manicure accessories**

EMULSIFYING AGENTS
BASF United Kingdom Ltd.
J. Bibby & Sons, Ltd.
Bio-Cosmetic Research
  Laboratories
Bush Boake Allen Ltd.,
  Perfumery Division
Rex Campbell & Co., Ltd.
Ciba Clayton Ltd.
Courtaulds Ltd.
Croda Ltd.
Cyclo Chemicals Ltd.
Dragoco (Gt. Britain) Ltd.
Dutton & Reinisch Ltd.
Fine Dyestuffs & Chemicals
  Ltd.
Food Industries Ltd.
Geigy (U.K.) Ltd.
Glovers (Chemicals) Ltd.
R. W. Greeff & Co., Ltd.
Guest Industrials Ltd.
Hoechst Chemicals Ltd.
Honeywill & Stein Ltd.
Honeywill-Atlas Ltd.
Howards of Ilford Ltd.
Imperial Chemical Industries
  Ltd.
Jacobson Van Den Berg & Co.
  (U.K.), Ltd.
Keegan Dystuffs & Chemicals
  Ltd.
Lankro Chemicals Ltd.
Leek Chemicals Ltd.
Lennig Chemicals Ltd.
Marchon Products Ltd.
L. E. Pritchitt & Co., Ltd.
Ronsheim & Moore Ltd.
Sandoz Products Ltd.
Shell Chemical U.K. Ltd.
Sipon Products Ltd.
Union Carbide Ltd.
  (Chemicals Division)
White Sea & Baltic Co. P. & I.
  Danischewsky Ltd.
Wilson & Mansfield Ltd.
Victor Wolf Ltd.

EOSOL
Croda Ltd.

**ESSENCE,
MOTHER-O'-PEARL**
Brown & Forth Ltd.
Rex Campbell & Co., Ltd.
Kingsley & Keith (Chemicals)
 Ltd.
May & Baker Ltd.
Shearman & Co., Ltd.
Alfred Paul White & Son

**ESSENTIAL OILS,
GENERAL**
Atkins & Co.
V. Berg & Sons, Ltd.
Bertrand Freres Ltd.
Blyth, Greene, Jourdain & Co.,
 Ltd.
Bruce, Starke & Co., Ltd.
Bush Boake Allen Ltd.,
 Perfumery Division
Charabot & Cie Ltd.
Antoine Chiris Ltd.
Cocker Chemical Co., Ltd.
F. D. Copeland & Sons, Ltd.
H. E. Daniel Ltd.
Dragoco (Gt. Britain) Ltd.
Dubuis & Rowsell Ltd.
Felton Company (Great
 Britain) Ltd.
Field & Co. (Aromatics), Ltd.
N.V. Chemische Fabriek Flebo
Food Industries Ltd.
H. Frischmann
Fuerst Day Lawson Ltd.
Gale & Mount Ltd.
A. J. Gomiero Ltd. (V. Mane
 Fils S.A.)
F. Gutkind & Co., Ltd.
Haarman & Reimer Ltd.
T. Harrison & Co., Ltd.
A. G. Hersom
M. Agusti Hidalgo (London)
 Ltd.
W. H. Hobbs & Co., Ltd.
Hollander Hyams Ltd.
Hollands Distillery (Essential
 Oils) Ltd.
Jacobson Van Den Berg & Co.
 (U.K.) Ltd.
John Kellys (London) Ltd.
Lautier Fils Ltd.
Gerald McDonald & Co., Ltd.
McVittie, Anderson & Co. Ltd.
J. & G. Miller
A. W. Munns & Co., Ltd.

Trade Agents for Mysore in
 London
'Naarden' (London) Ltd.
Natural & Synthetic
 Perfumery Essence Co.
Norda-Schimmel International
 Ltd.
P. T. Petley & Co., Ltd.
Pigalle (International) Ltd.
Roure Bertrand Fils et Justin
 Dupont
P. Samuelson & Co., Ltd.
R. Sarant & Co., Ltd.
Söflor Ltd.
Standard Synthetics Ltd.
Stevenson & Howell Ltd.
H. E. Stringer Ltd.
Techno Chemical Industries
 Ltd.
R. C. Treatt & Co., Ltd.
Alfred Paul White & Son
White, Tomkins & Courage
 Ltd.
Wilson & Mansfield Ltd.
Chas. Zimmermann & Co.,
 Ltd.

**ESSENTIAL OILS,
TERPENELESS**
Aromatica Ltd.
Bertrand Freres Ltd.
Bush Boake Allen Ltd.,
 Perfumery Division
Charabot & Cie Ltd.
Antoine Chiris Ltd.
Cocker Chemical Co., Ltd.
H. E. Daniel Ltd.
Dragoco (Gt. Britain) Ltd.
Dubuis & Rowsell Ltd.
Felton Company (Great
 Britain) Ltd.
Field & Co. (Aromatics), Ltd.
Firmenich Ltd.
Food Industries Ltd.
Fuerst Day Lawson Ltd.
Gale & Mount Ltd.
A. J. Gomiero Ltd. (V. Mane
 Fils S.A.)
F. Gutkind & Co., Ltd.
Haarman & Reimer Ltd.
T. Harrison & Co., Ltd.
M. Agusti Hidalgo (London)
 Ltd.
W. H. Hobbs & Co., Ltd.
Hollands Distillery (Essential
 Oils) Ltd.

International Flavours &
 Fragrances I.F.F. (Gt.
 Britain) Ltd.
Jacobson Van Den Berg & Co.
 (U.K.) Ltd.
Lanitis Bros. Ltd.
Lautier Fils Ltd.
Lockwood Magrath Pty., Ltd.
Gerald McDonald & Co., Ltd.
McVittie, Anderson & Co.,
 Ltd.
J. & G. Miller
A. W. Munns & Co., Ltd.
'Naarden' (London) Ltd.
Norda-Schimmel International
 Ltd.
P. T. Petley & Co., Ltd.
Pigalle (International) Ltd.
Roure Bertrand Fils et Justin
 Dupont
P. Samuelson & Co., Ltd.
R. Sarant & Co., Ltd.
Söflor Ltd.
Standard Synthetics Ltd.
Stevenson & Howell Ltd.
H. E. Stringer Ltd.
Supreme Mfg. Co., Ltd.
White, Tomkins & Courage
 Ltd.
Wilson & Mansfield Ltd.
Chas. Zimmermann & Co.,
 Ltd.

ETHYL ACETATE
Alcohols Ltd.
Barter Trading Corporation
 Ltd.
Bush Boake Allen Ltd.,
 Perfumery Division
Rex Campbell & Co., Ltd.
Food Industries Ltd.
The General Chemical Co.,
 Ltd.
Methylating Co., Ltd.

ETHYL ADIPATE
Dragoco (Gt. Britain) Ltd.

ETHYL LACTATE
Bowmans Chemicals Ltd.
Rex Campbell & Co., Ltd.
The General Chemical Co.,
 Ltd.
Howards of Ilford Ltd.
Tar Residuals Ltd.

ETHYLENEDIAMINE TETRA-ACETIC ACID (and Salts)
A.B.M. Industrial Products Ltd.
Allied Colloids Manufacturing Co., Ltd.
Bowmans Chemicals Ltd.
Geigy (U.K.) Ltd.
Sherman Chemicals Ltd.

ETHYLENE DICHLORIDE
The General Chemical Co., Ltd.
J. M. Steel & Co., Ltd.

ETHYLENE GLYCOL
BASF United Kingdom Ltd.
Rex Campbell & Co., Ltd.
The General Chemical Co., Ltd.
Hoechst Chemicals Ltd.
Honeywill & Stein Ltd.
Imperial Chemical Industries Ltd.
A. Revai & Co. (Chemicals) Ltd.
Shell Chemicals U.K. Ltd.
Sherman Chemicals Ltd.
Union Carbide Ltd. (Chemicals Division)

EUCALYPTUS OIL
V. Berg & Sons, Ltd.
Bertrand Freres Ltd.
Bruce, Starke & Co., Ltd.
Brush Boake Allen Ltd., Perfumery Division
Charabot & Cie Ltd.
F. D. Copeland & Sons, Ltd.
Courtin & Warner Ltd.
H. E. Daniel Ltd.
Food Industries Ltd.
Fuerst Day Lawson Ltd.
Gale & Mount Ltd.
A. J. Gomiero Ltd. (V. Mane Fils S.A.)
Geo. T. Gurr Ltd.
F. Gutkind & Co., Ltd.
T. Harrison & Co., Ltd.
A. G. Hersom
W. H. Hobbs & Co., Ltd.
Hollander Hyams Ltd.
Lautier Fils Ltd.
McVittie Anderson & Co., Ltd.
Norda-Schimmel International Ltd.
R. Sarant & Co., Ltd.

Standard Synthetics Ltd.
R. C. Treatt & Co., Ltd.
White, Tomkins & Courage Ltd.
Wilson & Mansfield Ltd.
Chas. Zimmermann & Co., Ltd.

EYELASH BRUSHES
Rene Heymans Ltd.
A. V. Pound & Co., Ltd.
Reeves & Sons, Ltd.

FACIAL CLEANSING TISSUES
Jeyes Group Ltd.
Kimberly-Clark Ltd.
Lambournes (Birmingham) Ltd.

FARINA
H. J. Evans & Co., Ltd.
Harry B. Wood Ltd.

FATTY ACIDS AND DERIVATIVES
See also under **Oleic, stearic, myristic,** *etc.*
Armour Hess Chemicals Ltd.
Bowring, Jones & Tidy Ltd.
Bush Boake Allen Ltd., Perfumery Division
Croda Ltd.
Dragoco (Gt. Britain) Ltd.
Durham Raw Materials Ltd.
Dutton & Reinisch Ltd.
Edipro Ltd.
R. W. Greeff & Co., Ltd.
M. Hamburger & Sons, Ltd.
Hercules Powder Co., Ltd.
Langley-Smith & Co., Ltd.
Leek Chemicals Ltd.
E. J. R. Lovelock
Meade-King Robinson & Co., Ltd.
Price's (Bromborough) Ltd.
Procter & Gamble Ltd.
Tar Residuals Ltd.
The Universal Oil Co., Ltd.
White Sea & Baltic Co. P. & I. Danischewsky Ltd.
Victor Wolf Ltd.
Wynmouth Lehr & Fatoils Ltd.

FERRIC CHLORIDE
BASF United Kingdom Ltd.
Berk Ltd.
British Anhydrous Ammonia Co., Ltd.

The General Chemical Co., Ltd.
Kingsley & Keith (Chemicals) Ltd.
Laporte Industries Ltd. (General Chemicals Division–Leeds)
L. R. B. Pearce Ltd.
Sherman Chemicals Ltd.
Tar Residuals Ltd.

FERRIC OXIDE (RED)
D. F. Anstead Ltd.
BASF United Kingdom Ltd.
British Anhydrous Ammonia Co., Ltd.
H. J. Evans & Co., Ltd.
Golden Valley Colours Ltd.
W. Hawley & Son, Ltd.
Howards of Ilford Ltd.
Laporte Industries Ltd. (Organics & Pigments Division–Ilford)
Thomas Morson & Son, Ltd.
Pfizer Ltd.
Procter, Johnson & Co., Ltd.
C. E. Ramsden & Co., Ltd.
Shearman & Co., Ltd.
J. M. Steel & Co., Ltd.
Williams (Hounslow) Ltd.

FERROUS SULPHIDE
H. J. Evans & Co., Ltd.
Laporte Industries Ltd. (General Chemicals Division–Leeds)
Sherman Chemicals Ltd.

FILTER CLOTH
Berk Ltd.
Robert Kellie & Son, Ltd.
Locker Industries Ltd.
Premier Filterpress Co., Ltd.
Townson & Mercer Ltd.
Turner Brothers Asbestos Co., Ltd.

FILTER PAPER
J. Barcham Green Ltd.
Carlson-Ford Sales Ltd.
A. Gallenkamp & Co., Ltd.
The General Chemical Co., Ltd.
Hospital & Laboratory Supplies Ltd.
S. H. Johnson & Co., Ltd.
Scientific Glass-Blowing Co.
Technical Paper Sales Ltd.
Townson & Mercer Ltd.

FLAVOURS

Bertrand Freres Ltd.
H. E. Daniel Ltd.
Dragoco (Gt. Britain) Ltd.
Dubuis & Rowsell Ltd.
Firmenich Ltd.
Florasynth Ltd.
Food Industries Ltd.
Fuerst Day Lawson Ltd.
Gale & Mount Ltd.
A. J. Gomiero Ltd. (V. Mane Fils S.A.)
Haarman & Reimer Ltd.
T. Harrison & Co., Ltd.
W. H. Hobbs & Co., Ltd.
International Flavours & Fragrances I.F.F. (Gt. Britain) Ltd.
Lautier Fils Ltd.
Lockwood, Magrath Pty., Ltd.
'Naarden' (London) Ltd.
Norda-Schimmel International Ltd.
P. T. Petley & Co., Ltd.
Pigalle (International) Ltd.
R. Sarant & Co., Ltd.
Scottish Flavour & Colour Co., Ltd.
Söflor Ltd.
Stevenson & Howell Ltd.
H. E. Stringer Ltd.
Supreme Mfg. Co., Ltd.
R. C. Treatt & Co., Ltd.
White, Tomkins & Courage Ltd.
Chas. Zimmermann & Co., Ltd.

FORMALDEHYDE

Barter Trading Corporation Ltd.
BASF United Kingdom Ltd.
Berk Ltd.
Rex Campbell & Co., Ltd.
Ciba Clayton Ltd.
The General Chemical Co., Ltd.
James Greenshields & Co., Ltd.
Geo. T. Gurr Ltd.
May & Baker Ltd.
Millwards Merchandise Ltd.
Sherman Chemicals Ltd.
J. M. Steel & Co., Ltd.
Synthite Ltd.
Tar Residuals Ltd.
Walker Chemical Co., Ltd.
Harry B. Wood Ltd.

A. & M. Zimmermann

FULLER'S EARTH

Berk Ltd.
Fullers' Earth Union Ltd.

GELATINE

Cheshire Gelatines
T. M. Duché & Sons (U.K.), Ltd.
Food Industries Ltd.
Edward Gorton Ltd. (Cheshire Gelatines Branch)
F. Gutkind & Co., Ltd.
Supreme Mfg. Co., Ltd.
Union Glue & Gelatine Co., Ltd.
A. & M. Zimmermann

GELLING AGENTS

Berk Ltd.
British Celanese Ltd.
Bush Beach & Segner Bayley Ltd.
J. W. Cumming & Son, Ltd.
Fine Dyestuffs & Chemicals Ltd.
Glovers (Chemicals) Ltd.
F. Gutkind & Co., Ltd.
Hardman & Holden Ltd.
Honeywill & Stein Ltd.
Victor Wolf Ltd.

GERANIUM OILS

V. Berg & Sons, Ltd.
Bertrand Freres Ltd.
Blyth, Greene, Jourdain & Co., Ltd.
Bush Boake Allen Ltd., Perfumery Division
Charabot & Cie Ltd.
Antoine Chiris Ltd.
F. D. Copeland & Sons, Ltd.
H. E. Daniel Ltd.
Dragoco (Gt. Britain) Ltd.
Fuerst Day Lawson Ltd.
Gale & Mount Ltd.
A. J. Gomiero Ltd. (V. Mane Fils S.A.)
F. Gutkind & Co., Ltd.
A. G. Hersom
W. H. Hobbs & Co., Ltd.
Hollander Hyams Ltd.
Lautier Fils Ltd.
Mallagh & Co.
McVittie Anderson & Co., Ltd.
A. W. Munns & Co., Ltd.

Natural & Synthetic Perfumery Essence Co.
Norda-Schimmel International Ltd.
P. Robertet & Cie
Roure Bertrand Fils et Justin Dupont
P. Samuelson & Co., Ltd.
R. Sarant & Co., Ltd.
Söflor Ltd.
Standard Synthetics Ltd.
H. E. Stringer Ltd.
R. C. Treatt & Co., Ltd.
Wilson & Mansfield Ltd.
Chas. Zimmermann & Co., Ltd.

GLUCOSE

Corn Products (Sales) Ltd.
Food Industries Ltd.
Laing-National Ltd.

GLYCERIN

Fredk. Boehm Ltd.
W. M. Delf (Liverpool) Ltd.
Food Industries Ltd.
Fuerst Day Lawson Ltd.
Gerard-Polysulphin Ltd.
Glycerine Ltd.
E. J. R. Lovelock
Thomas Morson & Son, Ltd.
'Naarden' (London) Ltd.
Procter & Gamble Ltd.
Sherman Chemicals Ltd.
The Universal Oil Co., Ltd.
Victor Wolf Ltd.
Wynmouth Lehr & Fatoils Ltd.

GLYCERIN SUBSTITUTES

Hoechst Chemicals Ltd.
Imperial Chemical Industries Ltd.

GLYCERYL DIACETATE

Bush Boake Allen Ltd., Perfumery Division
Rex Campbell & Co., Ltd.
Leek Chemicals Ltd.

GLYCERYL MONO-STEARATE

See under **Emulsifying agents**

GLYCOL STEARATE

See under **Emulsifying agents**

GUAIACOL

Bush Boake Allen Ltd., Perfumery Division

Hollander Hyams Ltd.
Sherman Chemicals Ltd.

GUM TRAGACANTH
V. Berg & Sons, Ltd.
Berk Ltd.
Brown & Forth Ltd.
Bush Boake Allen Ltd.,
  Perfumery Division
J. W. Cumming & Son, Ltd.
H. E. Daniel Ltd.
T. M. Duché & Sons (U.K.),
  Ltd.
Ellis Jones & Co. (Stockport),
  Ltd.
Food Industries Ltd.
H. Frischmann
Fuerst Day Lawson Ltd.
M. Hamburger & Sons, Ltd.
Impag (London) Ltd.
H. Lattimer
Millwards Merchandise Ltd.
Supreme Mfg. Co., Ltd.
Thew Arnott & Co., Ltd.

GUMS, GENERAL
Berk Ltd.
Bertrand Freres Ltd.
British Celanese Ltd.
Bush Boake Allen Ltd.,
  Perfumery Division
Courtaulds Ltd.
J. W. Cumming & Son, Ltd.
H. E. Daniel Ltd.
T. M. Duché & Sons (U.K.),
  Ltd.
Ellis Jones & Co. (Stockport),
  Ltd.
Joseph Flach & Sons, Ltd.
Food Industries Ltd.
H. Frischmann
Fuerst Day Lawson Ltd.
F. Gutkind & Co., Ltd.
M. Hamburger & Sons, Ltd.
Hollander Hyams Ltd.
Impag (London) Ltd.
John Kellys (London) Ltd.
H. Lattimer
Millwards Merchandise Ltd.
R. Sarant & Co., Ltd.
Shearman & Co., Ltd.
Sichel Adhesives Ltd.
Supreme Mfg. Co., Ltd.
Thew, Arnott & Co., Ltd.

**HENNA, HENNA
COMPOUNDS, etc.**
Joseph Flach & Sons, Ltd.
John Kellys (London) Ltd.

HEXYLENE GLYCOL
Barter Trading Corporation
  Ltd.
Methylating Co., Ltd.
Shell Chemicals U.K. Ltd.

HUON PINE OIL
White Sea & Baltic Co. P. & I.
  Danischewsky Ltd.

HYDROGEN PEROXIDE
Alcock (Peroxide) Ltd.
Berk Ltd.
Brown & Forth Ltd.
Cyclo Chemicals Ltd.
The General Chemical Co.,
  Ltd.
Keegan Dyestuffs & Chemicals
  Ltd.
Laporte Industries Ltd.
  (General Chemicals
  Division–Luton)
Millwards Merchandise Ltd.
Thomas Morson & Son, Ltd.

**HYDROGEN PEROXIDE
'SOLID'**
Laporte Industries Ltd.
  (General Chemicals
  Division–Luton)

**HYDROXY BENZOIC
ACID ESTERS**
Guest Industrials Ltd.
Nipa Laboratories Ltd.

**ICHTHAMMOL
(ICHTHYOL)**
Norda-Schimmel International
  Ltd.
A. Revai & Co. (Chemicals),
  Ltd.
Chas. Zimmermann & Co.,
  Ltd.

IRISH MOSS
See **'Carragheen Moss'**

IRON SULPHATE
British Anhydrous Ammonia
  Co., Ltd.
British Titan Products Co.,
  Ltd.
East Lancashire Chemical Co.,
  Ltd.
H. J. Evans & Co., Ltd.
The General Chemical Co.,
  Ltd.
Harrison, Clark Ltd.
Jessop & Co.

Kingsley & Keith (Chemicals)
  Ltd.
Thomas Morson & Son, Ltd.
Procter, Johnson & Co., Ltd.
Shearman & Co., Ltd.
Sherman Chemicals Ltd.
A. & M. Zimmermann

IRON SULPHIDE
See **Ferrous sulphide**

ISOBORNEOL
Victor Blagden & Co., Ltd.
H. E. Daniel Ltd.
Dragoco (Gt. Britain) Ltd.
Kingsley & Keith (Chemicals)
  Ltd.
Natural & Synthetic Perfumery
  Essence Co.

ISO-JASMONES
Dragoco (Gt. Britain) Ltd.
Firmenich Ltd.
Givaudan & Co., Ltd.
A. W. Munns & Co., Ltd.
Natural & Synthetic Perfumery
  Essence Co.
Roure Bertrand Fils et Justin
  Dupont
P. Samuelson & Co., Ltd.

ISOPROPYL MYRISTATE
(*Also* **Isopropyl Palmitate-
Stearate**)
Barter Trading Corporation
  Ltd.
Bush Boake Allen Ltd.,
  Perfumery Division
Rex Campbell & Co., Ltd.
Croda Ltd.
Givaudan & Co., Ltd.
Leek Chemicals Ltd.

JASMINE ABSOLUTE
Bertrand Freres Ltd.
Bush Boake Allen Ltd.,
  Perfumery Division
Charabot & Cie Ltd.
Antoine Chiris Ltd.
F. D. Copeland & Sons, Ltd.
Dubuis & Rowsell Ltd.
A. J. Gomiero Ltd. (V. Mane
  Fils S.A.)
H. M. Langton & Co., Ltd.
Lautier Fils Ltd.
A. W. Munns & Co., Ltd.
Natural & Synthetic Perfumery
Essence Co.

Norda-Schimmel International
Ltd.
Roure Bertrand Fils et Justin
Dupont
P. Samuelson & Co., Ltd.
R. Sarant & Co., Ltd.
H. E. Stringer Ltd.
Alfred Paul White & Son
Wilson & Mansfield Ltd.

JASMONE
See **Iso-jasmones**

KAOLIN
See also **China clay** *and*
Colloidal clays
Richard Baker & Co., Ltd.
Berk Ltd.
Durham Raw Materials Ltd.
English Clays Lovering Pochin
& Co., Ltd.
H. J. Evans & Co., Ltd.
H. Lattimer
A. Levermore & Co., Ltd.
Thomas Morson & Son, Ltd.
New Consolidated Mines of
Cornwall Ltd.
Shearman & Co., Ltd.
Zach Cartwright Ltd.

KIESELGUHR
Richard Baker & Co., Ltd.
Berk Ltd.
H. J. Evans & Co., Ltd.
Johns-Manville (Gt. Britain)
Ltd.
William Kenyon & Sons
(Thermal Insulations), Ltd.
Thomas Morson & Son, Ltd.
Shearman & Co., Ltd.

LANOLIN
Croda Ltd.
Cyclo Chemicals Ltd.
Fuerst Day Lawson Ltd.
M. Hamburger & Sons, Ltd.
Jacobson Van Den Berg & Co.
(U.K.), Ltd.
E. J. R. Lovelock
Meade-King Robinson & Co.,
Ltd.
Pharmaceutical Lanoline Co.
Westbrook Lanolin Co.
(Woolcombers), Ltd.
Wynmouth Lehr & Fatoils Ltd.

LANOLIN DERIVATIVES
D. F. Anstead Ltd.
Croda Ltd.

Cyclo Chemicals Ltd.
Dutton & Reinisch Ltd.
M. Hamburger & Sons, Ltd.
Jacobson Van Den Berg & Co.
(U.K.), Ltd.
Kingsley & Keith (Chemicals)
Ltd.
Westbrook Lanolin Co.
(Woolcombers), Ltd.

LAVANDIN OIL
Bertrand Freres Ltd.
Bush Boake Allen Ltd.,
Perfumery Division
Charabot & Cie Ltd.
Antoine Chiris Ltd.
F. D. Copeland & Sons, Ltd.
Courtin & Warner Ltd.
H. E. Daniel Ltd.
Dragoco (Gt. Britain) Ltd.
Felton Company (Great
Britain) Ltd.
Fuerst Day Lawson Ltd.
Gale & Mount Ltd.
A. J. Gomiero Ltd. (V. Mane
Fils S.A.)
F. Gutkind & Co., Ltd.
A. G. Hersom
W. H. Hobbs & Co., Ltd.
Lautier Fils Ltd.
Mallagh & Co.
A. W. Munns & Co., Ltd.
Natural & Synthetic Perfumery
Essence Co.
Norda-Schimmel International
Ltd.
Pigalle (International) Ltd.
Roure Bertrand Fils et Justin
Dupont
P. Samuelson & Co., Ltd.
R. Sarant & Co., Ltd.
Söflor Ltd.
Standard Synthetics Ltd.
H. E. Stringer Ltd.
R. C. Treatt & Co., Ltd.
Alfred Paul White & Son
Wilson & Mansfield Ltd.
Chas. Zimmermann & Co.,
Ltd.

LAVENDER OIL
(ENGLISH)
Atkins & Co.
Bush Boake Allen Ltd.,
Perfumery Division
Dubuis & Rowsell Ltd.
Fuerst Day Lawson Ltd.
Lautier Fils Ltd.

William Ransom & Son, Ltd.
Söflor Ltd.
Standard Synthetics Ltd.

LAVENDER OIL
(FRENCH)
Bertrand Freres Ltd.
Bush Boake Allen Ltd.,
Perfumery Division
Charabot & Cie Ltd.
Antoine Chiris Ltd.
F. D. Copeland & Sons, Ltd.
Courtin & Warner Ltd.
H. E. Daniel Ltd.
Felton Company (Great
Britain) Ltd.
Fuerst Day Lawson Ltd.
Gale & Mount Ltd.
A. J. Gomiero Ltd. (V. Mane
Fils S.A.)
F. Gutkind & Co., Ltd.
A. G. Hersom
W. H. Hobbs & Co., Ltd.
Laboratoire Noel
Lautier Fils Ltd.
A. W. Munns & Co., Ltd.
Natural & Synthetic Perfumery
Essence Co.
Norda-Schimmel International
Ltd.
Pigalle (International) Ltd.
Roure Bertrand Fils et Justin
Dupont
P. Samuelson & Co., Ltd.
R. Sarant & Co., Ltd.
Söflor Ltd.
Standard Synthetics Ltd.
H. E. Stringer Ltd.
R. C. Treatt & Co., Ltd.
Alfred Paul White & Son
Wilson & Mansfield Ltd.
Chas. Zimmermann & Co.,
Ltd.

LECITHIN
D. F. Anstead Ltd.
Bio-Cosmetic Research
Laboratories
Fredk. Boehm Ltd.
British Oil & Cake Mills Ltd.
T. M. Duché & Sons (U.K.),
Ltd.
Kingsley & Keith (Chemicals)
Ltd.
E. J. R. Lovelock
L. E. Pritchitt & Co., Ltd.
A. Revai & Co. (Chemicals),
Ltd.

Wilson & Mansfield Ltd.
Wynmouth Lehr & Fatoils Ltd.

LEMON OIL
Bertrand Freres Ltd.
Bruce, Starke & Co., Ltd.
Bush Boake Allen Ltd.,
  Perfumery Division
Charabot & Cie Ltd.
Cocker Chemical Co., Ltd.
F. D. Copeland & Sons, Ltd.
Courtin & Warner Ltd.
H. E. Daniel Ltd.
Dragoco (Gt. Britain) Ltd.
Dubuis & Rowsell Ltd.
Felton Company (Great
  Britain) Ltd.
Food Industries Ltd.
Fuerst Day Lawson Ltd.
Gale & Mount Ltd.
A. J. Gomiero Ltd. (V. Mane
  Fils S.A.)
F. Gutkind & Co., Ltd.
T. Harrison & Co., Ltd.
A. G. Hersom
M. Agusti Hidalgo (London)
  Ltd.
W. H. Hobbs & Co., Ltd.
Hollander Hyams Ltd.
Lanitis Bros., Ltd.
Lockwood Magrath Pty., Ltd.
Mallagh & Co.
Gerald McDonald & Co., Ltd.
McVittie Anderson & Co., Ltd.
A. W. Munns & Co., Ltd.
Natural & Synthetic Perfumery
  Essence Co.
Norda-Schimmel International
  Ltd.
Pigalle (International) Ltd.
Roure Bertrand Fils et Justin
  Dupont
H. Rubeck Ltd.
P. Samuelson & Co., Ltd.
R. Sarant & Co., Ltd.
Sôflor Ltd.
Stevenson & Howell Ltd.
H. E. Stringer Ltd.
R. C. Treatt & Co., Ltd.
Alfred Paul White & Son
Wilson & Mansfield Ltd.
White, Tomkins & Courage
  Ltd.
Chas. Zimmermann & Co.,
  Ltd.

LEMONGRASS OIL
V. Berg & Sons, Ltd.

Blyth, Greene, Jourdain & Co.,
  Ltd.
Bush Boake Allen Ltd.,
  Perfumery Division
Charabot & Cie Ltd.
Courtin & Warner Ltd.
H. E. Daniel Ltd.
Felton Company (Great
  Britain), Ltd.
Food Industries Ltd.
Fuerst Day Lawson Ltd.
Gale & Mount Ltd.
A. G. Hersom
W. H. Hobbs & Co., Ltd.
John Kellys (London) Ltd.
Lautier Fils Ltd.
A. W. Munns & Co., Ltd.
Norda-Schimmel International
  Ltd.
Roure Bertrand Fils et Justin
  Dupont
R. Sarant & Co., Ltd.
R. C. Treatt & Co., Ltd.
White, Tomkins & Courage
  Ltd.
Wilson & Mansfield Ltd.
Chas. Zimmermann & Co.,
  Ltd.

LIME OIL
Bush Boake Allen Ltd.,
  Perfumery Division
Cocker Chemical Co., Ltd.
F. D. Copeland & Sons, Ltd.
H. E. Daniel Ltd.
Dubuis & Rowsell Ltd.
Felton Company (Great
  Britain) Ltd.
Food Industries Ltd.
Fuerst Day Lawson Ltd.
Gale & Mount Ltd.
A. J. Gomiero Ltd. (V. Mane
  Fils S.A.)
F. Gutkind & Co., Ltd.
A. G. Hersom
W. H. Hobbs & Co., Ltd.
Lautier Fils Ltd.
Gerald McDonald & Co., Ltd.
McVittie Anderson & Co., Ltd.
A. W. Munns & Co., Ltd.
P. Robertet & Cie
Roure Bertrand Fils et Justin
  Dupont
H. Rubeck Ltd.
P. Samuelson & Co., Ltd.
R. Sarant & Co., Ltd.
Sôflor Ltd.

Standard Synthetics Ltd.
Stevenson & Howell Ltd.
R. C. Treatt & Co., Ltd.
White, Tomkins & Courage
  Ltd.
Wilson & Mansfield Ltd.
Chas. Zimmermann & Co.,
  Ltd.

LINALOOL, SYNTHETIC
Bush Boake Allen Ltd.,
  Perfumery Division
Gale & Mount Ltd.
A. W. Munns & Co., Ltd.
Roche Products Ltd.
Standard Synthetics Ltd.
Chas. Zimmermann & Co.,
  Ltd.
*For natural sources of linalool,
see also under* **Essential oils**
and **Aromatic chemicals**

LINALYL ACETATE, SYNTHETIC
Bush Boake Allen Ltd.,
  Perfumery Division
Charabot & Cie Ltd.
Gale & Mount Ltd.
A. W. Munns & Co., Ltd.
Roche Products Ltd.
Sôflor Ltd.
Standard Synthetics Ltd.
Chas. Zimmermann & Co.,
  Ltd.
*For natural sources of linalyl
see also under* **Essential oils**
and **Aromatic chemicals**

LINOLEATES
D. F. Anstead Ltd.
Rex Campbell & Co., Ltd.
Leek Chemicals Ltd.
Price's (Bromborough) Ltd.
Victor Wolf Ltd.

LIP BRUSHES
Percy P. Baker Ltd.
Cope Allman Packaging
Rene Heymans Ltd.
A. V. Pound & Co., Ltd.

LIPSTICK CASES
All Metal Smallware Ltd.
Betts & Co., Ltd.
B. L. Engineering Co.
Blewis & Shaw (Plastics) Ltd.
Cope Allman Packaging
Motivity
H. G. Sanders & Sons, Ltd.

183

LIPSTICK DYESTUFF SOLVENTS
Dutton & Reinisch Ltd.

LIQUID PARAFFIN
See **Oils, mineral**

LITHOPONE
H. J. Evans & Co., Ltd.
Stanley G. Walker & Co., Ltd.

LYCOPODIUM
Berk Ltd.
Joseph Flach & Sons, Ltd.
H. Frischmann
The General Chemical Co.,
Ltd.

**MAGNESIUM
(METALLIC POWDER)**
Blackwell's Metallurgical
Works Ltd.

**MAGNESIUM
CARBONATE**
Chemical & Insulating Co.,
Ltd.
Dunn Bros. Manchester Ltd.
H. J. Evans & Co., Ltd.
The General Chemical Co.,
Ltd.
Howards of Ilford Ltd.
Kingsley & Keith (Chemicals)
Ltd.
Thomas Morson & Son, Ltd.
Newalls Insulation & Chemical
Co., Ltd.
Shearman & Co., Ltd.
Sherman Chemicals Ltd.

MAGNESIUM OXIDE
Chemical & Insulating Co.,
Ltd.
Dunn Bros. Manchester Ltd.
The General Chemical Co.,
Ltd.
R. W. Greeff & Co., Ltd.
Howards of Ilford Ltd.
Thomas Morson & Son, Ltd.
Newalls Insulation & Chemical
Co., Ltd.
C. E. Ramsden & Co., Ltd.
Shearman & Co., Ltd.
Sherman Chemicals Ltd.

**MAGNESIUM
PEROXIDE**
Laporte Industries Ltd.
(General Chemicals
Division–Luton)

MAGNESIUM STEARATE
See under **Stearates**

**MAGNESIUM SULPHATE
(Epsom Salts)**
Berk Ltd.
W. Blythe & Co., Ltd.
H. J. Evans & Co., Ltd.
Harris Hart & Co., Ltd.
Howards of Ilford Ltd.
Millwards Merchandise Ltd.
Tar Residuals Ltd.

**MANICURE
ACCESSORIES**
Osborne Garrett & Nagele Ltd.

MASCARA BRUSHES
Percy P. Baker Ltd.
Rene Heymans Ltd.

MENTHOL
V. Berg & Sons, Ltd.
Bertrand Freres Ltd.
Blyth, Greene, Jourdain & Co.,
Ltd.
Bush Boake Allen Ltd.,
Perfumery Division
Charabot & Cie Ltd.
H. E. Daniel Ltd.
Dragoco (Gt. Britain) Ltd.
Felton Company (Great
Britain) Ltd.
Food Industries Ltd.
H. Frischmann
Fuerst Day Lawson Ltd.
Gale & Mount Ltd.
A. J. Gomiero Ltd. (V. Mane
Fils S.A.)
Geo. T. Gurr Ltd.
F. Gutkind & Co., Ltd.
A. G. Hersom
W. H. Hobbs & Co., Ltd.
John Kellys (London) Ltd.
Lautier Fils Ltd.
McVittie Anderson & Co., Ltd.
A. W. Munns & Co., Ltd.
Roure Bertrand Fils et Justin
Dupont
R. Sarant & Co., Ltd.
R. C. Treatt & Co., Ltd.
Wilson & Mansfield Ltd.
Chas. Zimmermann & Co.,
Ltd.

METHYL ACETATE
Barter Trading Corporation
Ltd.
Rex Campbell & Co., Ltd.

The General Chemical Co.,
Ltd.
Methylating Co., Ltd.
J. M. Steel & Co., Ltd.

**METHYL NONYL
KETONE**
Gale & Mount Ltd.
Givaudan & Co., Ltd.
International Flavours &
Fragrances I.F.F. (Gt.
Britain) Ltd.
A. W. Munns & Co., Ltd.

METHYLATED SPIRIT
See **Alcohol (I.M.S.)**

**MICROCRYSTALLINE
WAXES**
See Under **Waxes**

MIMOSA ABSOLUTE
Bertrand Freres Ltd.
Bush Boake Allen Ltd.,
Perfumery Division
Charabot & Cie Ltd.
Antoine Chiris Ltd.
F. D. Copeland & Sons, Ltd.
A. J. Gomiero Ltd. (V. Mane
Fils S.A.)
Lautier Fils Ltd.
A. W. Munns & Co., Ltd.
Natural & Synthetic Perfumery
Essence Co.
Roure Bertrand Fils et Justin
Dupont
P. Samuelson & Co., Ltd.
R. Sarant & Co., Ltd.
H. E. Stringer Ltd.
Alfred Paul White & Son
Wilson & Mansfield Ltd.

MURIATIC ACID
See **Acid, hydrochloric**

MUSK
See also under **Perfumery
compounds**
V. Berg & Sons, Ltd.
Bertrand Freres Ltd.
Victor Blagden & Co., Ltd.
A. W. Munns & Co., Ltd.
Roure Bertrand Fils et Justin
Dupont
P. Samuelson & Co., Ltd.
Standard Synthetics Ltd.
R. C. Treatt & Co., Ltd.
Alfred Paul White & Son

MUSKS (Indane)
Firmenich Ltd.
Givaudan & Co., Ltd.
International Flavours &
  Fragrances I.F.F. (Gt.
  Britain) Ltd.
Söflor Ltd.

MUSKS (Macrocylic)
Victor Blagden & Co., Ltd.
Dragoco (Gt. Britain) Ltd.
Firmenich Ltd.
Gale & Mount Ltd.
Givaudan & Co., Ltd.
A. W. Munns & Co., Ltd.
Natural & Synthetic Perfumery
  Essence Co.
Wilson & Mansfield Ltd.

MUSKS (Nitro)
Bush Boake Allen Ltd.,
  Perfumery Division
Gale & Mount Ltd.
Givaudan & Co., Ltd.
Haarman & Reimer Ltd.
International Flavours &
  Fragrances I.F.F. (Gt.
  Britain) Ltd.
Natural & Synthetic Perfumery
  Essence Co.
Standard Synthetics Ltd.

MUSKS (Tetralin)
Givaudan & Co., Ltd.
W. H. Hobbs & Co., Ltd.
Söflor Ltd.

NAPHTHA
Anglo-Scottish Chemical Co.,
  Ltd.
The General Chemical Co.,
  Ltd.
Lancashire Tar Distillers Ltd.
London Tar & Chemical Co.,
  Ltd.
Midland Tar Distillers Ltd.
Scottish Tar Distillers Ltd.
Tar Residuals Ltd.
United Coke & Chemicals Co.,
  Ltd.

NAPHTHALENE
Anglo-Scottish Chemical Co.,
  Ltd.
The General Chemical Co.,
  Ltd.
Lancashire Tar Distillers Ltd.
London Tar & Chemical Co.,
  Ltd.

Midland Tar Distillers Ltd.
Scottish Tar Distillers Ltd.
Tar Residuals Ltd.
United Coke & Chemicals Co.,
  Ltd.
The United Steel Companies
  Ltd.
A. & M. Zimmermann

NAPHTHALENE
(REFINED)
Anglo-Scottish Chemical Co.,
  Ltd.
The General Chemical Co.,
  Ltd.
James Greenshields & Co., Ltd.
Jessop & Co.
Lancashire Tar Distillers Ltd.
Procter, Johnson & Co., Ltd.

NATURAL FLOWER
ABSOLUTES
Bertrand Freres Ltd.
Bush Boake Allen Ltd.,
  Perfumery Division
Charabot & Cie Ltd.
Dragoco (Gt. Britain) Ltd.
A. J. Gomiero Ltd. (V. Mane
  Fils S.A.)
Lautier Fils Ltd.
H. M. Langton & Co., Ltd.
Natural & Synthetic Perfumery
  Essence Co.
Norda-Schimmel International
  Ltd.
Pigalle (International) Ltd.
Roure Bertrand Fils et Justin
  Dupont
P. Samuelson & Co., Ltd.
Söflor Ltd.
H. E. Stringer Ltd.
Alfred Paul White & Son
Wilson & Mansfield Ltd.

NEOSYL
See under **Silica, amorphous**

NEROLI OIL
Bertrand Freres Ltd.
Bush Boake Allen Ltd.,
  Perfumery Division
Rex Campbell & Co., Ltd.
Charabot & Cie Ltd.
Antoine Chiris Ltd.
F. D. Copeland & Sons, Ltd.
H. E. Daniel Ltd.
Dragoco (Gt. Britain) Ltd.
Dubuis & Rowsell Ltd.

Felton Company (Great
  Britain) Ltd.
Fuerst Day Lawson Ltd.
Gale & Mount Ltd.
A. J. Gomiero Ltd. (V. Mane
  Fils S.A.)
W. H. Hobbs & Co., Ltd.
H. M. Langton & Co., Ltd.
Lautier Fils Ltd.
Mallagh & Co.
A. W. Munns & Co., Ltd.
Natural & Synthetic Perfumery
  Essence Co.
Norda-Schimmel International
  Ltd.
Pigalle (International) Ltd.
Roure Bertrand Fils et Justin
  Dupont
P. Samuelson & Co., Ltd.
R. Sarant & Co., Ltd.
Söflor Ltd.
H. E. Stringer Ltd.
R. C. Treatt & Co., Ltd.
Alfred Paul White & Son
Wilson & Mansfield Ltd.
Chas. Zimmermann & Co.,
  Ltd.

NIGROSINE
Butterfield Laboratories Ltd.
Ciba Clayton Ltd.
Williams (Hounslow) Ltd.
A. & M. Zimmermann

NUTMEG OIL
V. Berg & Sons, Ltd.
Bertrand Freres Ltd.
Blyth, Greene, Jourdain & Co.,
  Ltd.
Bush Boake Allen Ltd.,
  Perfumery Division
Charabot & Cie Ltd.
H. E. Daniel Ltd.
Dragoco (Gt. Britain) Ltd.
Food Industries Ltd.
Fuerst Day Lawson Ltd.
Gale & Mount Ltd.
A. J. Gomiero Ltd. (V. Mane
  Fils S.A.)
F. Gutkind & Co., Ltd.
W. H. Hobbs & Co., Ltd.
Lautier Fils Ltd.
A. W. Munns & Co., Ltd.
Norda-Schimmel International
  Ltd.
R. Sarant & Co., Ltd.
Standard Synthetics Ltd.
H. E. Stringer Ltd.

185

R. C. Treatt & Co., Ltd.
Alfred Paul White & Son
White, Tomkins & Courage
  Ltd.
Wilson & Mansfield Ltd.
Chas. Zimmermann & Co.,
  Ltd.

OCHRE
D. F. Anstead Ltd.
Butterfield Laboratories Ltd.
Golden Valley Colours Ltd.
W. Hawley & Son, Ltd.
Procter, Johnson & Co., Ltd.
Shearman & Co., Ltd.
Westwood Macneill & Co., Ltd.
Williams (Hounslow) Ltd.

OIL, AVOCADO
Bio-Cosmetic Research
  Laboratories
Fuerst Day Lawson Ltd.
A. G. Hersom
'Naarden' (London) Ltd.
Pigalle (International) Ltd.
P. Samuelson & Co., Ltd.
Wilson & Mansfield Ltd.

OIL, BIRCH TAR
Bertrand Freres Ltd.
Bush Boake Allen Ltd.,
  Perfumery Division
Charabot & Cie Ltd.
H. E. Daniel Ltd.
Dragoco (Gt. Britain) Ltd.
Food Industries Ltd.
A. J. Gomiero Ltd. (V. Mane
  Fils S.A.)
W. H. Hobbs & Co., Ltd.
A. W. Munns & Co., Ltd.
Sherman Chemicals Ltd.
Standard Synthetics Ltd.
White Sea & Baltic Co.,
  P. & I. Danischewsky Ltd.

OIL, CARDAMON
H. E. Daniel Ltd.
Dragoco (Gt. Britain) Ltd.
Fuerst Day Lawson Ltd.
Gale & Mount Ltd.
A. W. Munns & Co., Ltd.
Natural & Synthetic Perfumery
  Essence Co.
Norda-Schimmel International
  Ltd.
Söflor Ltd.
H. E. Stringer Ltd.
Chas. Zimmermann & Co.,
  Ltd.

OIL, CASTOR
Bowring, Jones & Tidy Ltd.
S. Bramwell & Co., Ltd.
British Oil & Cake Mills Ltd.
Ellis Jones & Co. (Stockport),
  Ltd.
Fuerst Day Lawson Ltd.
Geo. T. Gurr Ltd.
M. Hamburger & Sons, Ltd.
E. J. R. Lovelock
Meade-King, Robinson & Co.,
  Ltd.
Millwards Merchandise Ltd.
Velho Blackstock & Co., Ltd.
A. & M. Zimmermann

OIL, CELERY
Bertrand Freres Ltd.
Charabot & Cie Ltd.
Antoine Chiris Ltd.
H. E. Daniel Ltd.
Dragoco (Gt. Britain) Ltd.
Gale & Mount Ltd.
A. J. Gomiero Ltd. (V. Mane
  Fils S.A.)
A. W. Munns & Co., Ltd.
Natural & Synthetic Perfumery
  Essence Co.
R. Sarant & Co., Ltd.
Standard Synthetics Ltd.
H. E. Stringer Ltd.
R. C. Treatt & Co., Ltd.
Alfred Paul White & Son
Chas. Zimmermann & Co.,
  Ltd.

OIL, COCONUT
J. Bibby & Sons, Ltd.
Bowring, Jones & Tidy Ltd.
S. Bramwell & Co., Ltd.
British Oil and Cake Mills Ltd.
Fuerst Day Lawson Ltd.
M. Hamburger & Sons, Ltd.
H. Lattimer
E. J. R. Lovelock
Meade-King Robinson & Co.
  Ltd.
Millwards Merchandise Ltd.
L. E. Pritchitt & Co., Ltd.
Procter & Gamble Ltd.
Velho Blackstock & Co., Ltd.

OIL, COTTONSEED
Bartoline (Hull) Ltd.
V. Berg & Sons, Ltd.
J. Bibby & Sons, Ltd.
Blyth, Greene, Jourdain & Co.,
  Ltd.

Bowring, Jones & Tidy Ltd.
S. Bramwell & Co., Ltd.
British Oil and Cake Mills Ltd.
F. Chiesman & Co., Ltd.
Fuerst Day Lawson Ltd.
M. Hamburger & Sons, Ltd.
E. J. R. Lovelock
Meade-King Robinson & Co.,
  Ltd.
Velho Blackstock & Co., Ltd.

OIL, CUBEB
H. E. Daniel Ltd.
Gale & Mount Ltd.
A. W. Munns & Co., Ltd.

OIL, DILL SEED
Courtin & Warner Ltd.
H. E. Daniel Ltd.
Dragoco (Gt. Britain) Ltd.
Fuerst Day Lawson Ltd.
Gale & Mount Ltd.
Norda-Schimmel International
  Ltd.
Standard Synthetics Ltd.
Alfred Paul White & Son
Wilson & Mansfield

OIL, GINGER
Charabot & Cie Ltd.
H. E. Daniel Ltd.
Dragoco (Gt. Britain) Ltd.
Fuerst Day Lawson Ltd.
Gale & Mount Ltd.
A. W. Munns & Co., Ltd.
Wm. Ransom & Son, Ltd.
R. C. Treatt & Co., Ltd.
Chas. Zimmermann & Co.,
  Ltd.

OIL, GRAPE SEED
Blyth, Greene, Jourdain & Co.,
  Ltd.
M. Agusti Hidalgo (London)
  Ltd.
E. J. R. Lovelock

OIL, LINSEED
Bartoline (Hull) Ltd.
Bowring, Jones & Tidy Ltd.
British Oil and Cake Mills Ltd.
Fuerst Day Lawson Ltd.
M. Hamburger & Sons, Ltd.
E. J. R. Lovelock
Meade-King Robinson & Co.,
  Ltd.
Velho Blackstock & Co., Ltd.

OIL, OLIVE

Astor Boisselier & Lawrence Ltd.
F. Chiesman & Co., Ltd.
Croda Ltd.
Food Industries Ltd.
Fuerst Day Lawson Ltd.
M. Hamburger & Sons, Ltd.
E. J. R. Lovelock

OIL, PARSLEY

Bertrand Freres Ltd.
Charabot & Cie Ltd.
H. E. Daniel Ltd.
Dragoco (Gt. Britain) Ltd.
Gale & Mount Ltd.
A. J. Gomiero Ltd. (V. Mane Fils S.A.)
A. W. Munns & Co., Ltd.
R. Sarant & Co., Ltd.
Söflor Ltd.
H. E. Stringer Ltd.
Alfred Paul White & Son
Wilson & Mansfield Ltd.
Chas. Zimmermann & Co., Ltd.

OIL, PEACH KERNEL

J. Bibby & Sons, Ltd.
Bush Boake Allen Ltd., Perfumery Division
Fuerst Day Lawson Ltd.
A. G. Hersom

OIL, PEPPER

Charabot & Cie Ltd.
H. E. Daniel Ltd.
Dragoco (Gt. Britain) Ltd.
Fuerst Day Lawson Ltd.
Gale & Mount Ltd.
A. J. Gomiero Ltd. (V. Mane Fils S.A.)
A. W. Munns & Co., Ltd.
R. Sarant & Co., Ltd.
Söflor Ltd.
Standard Synthetics Ltd.
Alfred Paul White & Son
Wilson & Mansfield Ltd.
Chas. Zimmermann & Co., Ltd.

OIL, PIMENTO BERRY

H. E. Daniel Ltd.
Fuerst Day Lawson Ltd.
Gale & Mount Ltd.
A. J. Gomiero Ltd. (V. Mane Fils S.A.)
A. W. Munns & Co., Ltd.
Standard Synthetics Ltd.

R. C. Treatt & Co., Ltd.

OIL, RAISIN (GRAPE) SEED

E. J. R. Lovelock

OIL, ROSIN

Hercules Powder Co., Ltd.
E. J. R. Lovelock
Meade-King, Robinson & Co., Ltd.
A. V. Pound & Co., Ltd.
Smith & Forrest (Oils) Ltd.
Tar Residuals Ltd.
Thew, Arnott & Co., Ltd.
Wynmouth Lehr & Fatoils Ltd.

OIL, SPEARMINT

F. D. Copeland & Sons, Ltd.
Courtin & Warner Ltd.
H. E. Daniel Ltd.
Dragoco (Gt. Britain) Ltd.
Fuerst Day Lawson Ltd.
Gale & Mount Ltd.
A. J. Gomiero Ltd. (V. Mane Fils S.A.)
Hollander Hyams Ltd.
John Kellys (London) Ltd.
Lautier Fils Ltd.
A. W. Munns & Co., Ltd.
Norda-Schimmel International Ltd.
P. T. Petley & Co., Ltd.
Söflor Ltd.
Standard Synthetics Ltd.
H. E. Stringer Ltd.
R. C. Treatt & Co., Ltd.
Wilson & Mansfield Ltd.
Chas. Zimmermann & Co., Ltd.

OIL, SWEET ALMOND

Courtin & Warner Ltd.
H. E. Daniel
Food Industries Ltd.
Gale & Mount Ltd.
F. Gutkind & Co., Ltd.
A. G. Hersom
A. W. Munns & Co., Ltd.
Söflor Ltd.
Wilson & Mansfield Ltd.
Chas. Zimmermann & Co., Ltd.

OIL, TEA SEED

V. Berg & Sons, Ltd.
Bowring, Jones & Tidy Ltd.
Velho Blackstock & Co., Ltd.

OIL, TI-TREE

Bush Boake Allen Ltd., Perfumery Division
H. E. Daniel Ltd.
Gale & Mount Ltd.
McVittie Anderson & Co., Ltd.
Standard Synthetics Ltd.
Wilson & Mansfield Ltd.

OIL, TURTLE

Blyth, Greene, Jourdain & Co., Ltd.
Fuerst Day Lawson Ltd.
M. Hamburger & Sons, Ltd.

OILS, FISH LIVER

Bartoline (Hull) Ltd.
E. J. R. Lovelock
Meade-King Robinson & Co., Ltd.
Velho Blackstock & Co., Ltd.

OILS, HALF-WHITE

See **Oils, mineral**

OILS, HYDROGENATED (GENERAL)

Armour Hess Chemicals Ltd.
J. Bibby & Sons, Ltd.
S. Bramwell & Co., Ltd.
British Oil & Cake Mills Ltd.
E. J. R. Lovelock
Mead-King Robinson & Co. Ltd.
Millwards Merchandise Ltd.
Pigalle (International) Ltd.
L. E. Pritchitt & Co., Ltd.
Procter & Gamble Ltd.

OILS, MARINE (GENERAL)

S. Bramwell & Co., Ltd.
British Oil and Cake Mills Ltd.
E. J. R. Lovelock
Meade-King, Robinson & Co., Ltd.
L. E. Pritchitt & Co., Ltd.
Procter & Gamble Ltd.
Velho Blackstock & Co., Ltd.

OILS, MINERAL

Astor Boisselier & Lawrence Ltd.
Henry Barlow & Sons (Oils), Ltd.
Burmah Oil Trading Ltd. Lobitos Division
Castrol Ltd.
Gulf Oil (Great Britain) Ltd.

Holroyd's Oil & Ceresine Co.,
Ltd.
Pharmaceutical Lanoline Co.
Purfinol Ltd.

OILS, PALM
V. Berg & Sons, Ltd.
J. Bibby & Sons, Ltd.
S. Bramwell & Co., Ltd.
British Oil & Cake Mills Ltd.
Fuerst Day Lawson Ltd.
M. Hamburger & Sons, Ltd.
H. Lattimer
E. J. R. Lovelock
Mead-King Robinson & Co.,
Ltd.
L. E. Pritchitt & Co., Ltd.
Procter & Gamble Ltd.
Velho, Blackstock & Co., Ltd.

OILS, PETROLEUM
See **Oils, mineral**

OILS, PINE
Bowring, Jones & Tidy Ltd.
Charabot & Cie Ltd.
Cocker Chemical Co., Ltd.
H. E. Daniel Ltd.
Dragoco (Gt. Britain) Ltd.
Fuerst Day Lawson Ltd.
Gale & Mount Ltd.
T. Harrison & Co., Ltd.
Hercules Powder Co., Ltd.
A. G. Hersom
W. H. Hobbs & Co., Ltd.
Kingsley & Keith (Chemicals)
Ltd.
Langley-Smith & Co., Ltd.
Meade-King Robinson & Co.,
Ltd.
A. W. Munns & Co., Ltd.
Norda-Schimmel International
Ltd.
A. V. Pound & Co., Ltd.
Wm. Ransome & Son, Ltd.
Roure Bertrand Fils et Justin
Dupont
R. Sarant & Co., Ltd.
Söflor Ltd.
Standard Synthetics Ltd.
Tar Residuals Ltd.
R. C. Treatt & Co., Ltd.
White Sea & Baltic Co.,
P. & I. Danischewsky Ltd.
Wynmouth Lehr & Fatoils Ltd.
A. & M. Zimmermann

OILS, SULPHONATED
Bowmans Chemicals Ltd.

Ciba Clayton Ltd.
East Lancashire Chemical Co.,
Ltd.
Ellis Jones & Co. (Stockport),
Ltd.
Esperis S.A.
Henkel International G.m.b.H.
Imperial Chemical Industries
Ltd.
Keegan Dyestuffs & Chemicals
Ltd.
Lankro Chemicals Ltd.
Meade-King Robinson & Co.,
Ltd.
Millwards Merchandise Ltd.
Velho Blackstock & Co., Ltd.

OILS, TURKEY RED
See **Oils, sulphonated**

OILS, WHITE
See under **Oils, mineral**

OLEATES
See suppliers of **Stearates**

OLEIC ACID
S. Bramwell & Co., Ltd.
Bush, Beach and Segner Bayley
Ltd.
Croda Ltd.
Cyclo Chemicals Ltd.
Durham Raw Materials Ltd.
The General Chemical Co.,
Ltd.
Henkel International G.m.b.H.
E. J. R. Lovelock
Meade-King, Robinson & Co.,
Ltd.
Millwards Merchandise Ltd.
Thomas Morson & Son, Ltd.
Price's (Bromborough) Ltd.
Techno Chemical Industries
J. C. Thompson & Co. (Duron),
Ltd.
Universal Oil Co., Ltd.
Victor Wolf Ltd.
Wynmouth Lehr & Fatoils Ltd.

ORANGE FLOWER
ABSOLUTE
Bertrand Freres Ltd.
Bush Boake Allen Ltd.,
Perfumery Division
Charabot & Cie Ltd.
F. D. Copeland & Sons, Ltd.
Dragoco (Gt. Britain) Ltd.
Dubuis & Rowsell Ltd.
Felton Co. (Great Britain),
Ltd.

Food Industries Ltd.
Lautier Fils Ltd.
A. W. Munns & Co., Ltd.
Natural & Synthetic Perfumery
Essence Co.
Norda-Schimmel International
Ltd.
Roure Bertrand Fils et Justin
Dupont
P. Samuelson & Co., Ltd.
R. Sarant & Co. Ltd.
Söflor Ltd.
H. E. Stringer Ltd.
Alfred Paul White & Son
Wilson & Mansfield Ltd.

ORANGE OIL
Bertrand Freres Ltd.
Bruce, Starke & Co., Ltd.
Bush Boake Allen Ltd.,
Perfumery Division
Charabot & Cie Ltd.
F. D. Copeland & Sons, Ltd.
H. E. Daniel Ltd.
Dragoco (Gt. Britain) Ltd.
Dubuis & Rowsell Ltd.
Felton Company (Great
Britain) Ltd.
Food Industries Ltd.
Fuerst Day Lawson Ltd.
Gale & Mount Ltd.
A. J. Gomiero Ltd. (V. Mane
Fils S.A.)
F. Gutkind & Co., Ltd.
T. Harrison & Co., Ltd.
A. G. Hersom
M. Agusti Hidalgo (London)
Ltd.
W. H. Hobbs & Co., Ltd.
Hollander Hyams Ltd.
Jacobson Van Den Berg & Co.
(U.K.), Ltd.
Lanitis Bros. Ltd.
Lautier Fils Ltd.
Lockwood, Magrath Pty., Ltd.
Gerald McDonald & Co., Ltd.
McVittie Anderson & Co., Ltd.
A. W. Munns & Co., Ltd.
Natural & Synthetic Perfumery
Essence Co.
Norda-Schimmel International
Ltd.
P. T. Petley & Co., Ltd.
Pigalle (International) Ltd.
Roure Bertrand Fils et Justin
Dupont
H. Rubeck Ltd.

P. Samuelson & Co.
R. Sarant & Co., Ltd.
Sōflor Ltd.
Stevenson and Howell Ltd.
H. E. Stringer Ltd.
Techno Chemical Industries Ltd.
R. C. Treatt & Co., Ltd.
Alfred Paul White & Son
White, Tomkins & Courage Ltd.
Wilson & Mansfield Ltd.
Chas. Zimmermann & Co., Ltd.

ORANGE STICKS
See **Manicure accessories**

ORRIS
Bertrand Freres Ltd.
Bush Boake Allen Ltd., Perfumery Division
Charabot & Cie Ltd.
Antoine Chiris Ltd.
H. E. Daniel Ltd.
Dragoco (Gt. Britain) Ltd.
Lautier Fils Ltd.
Joseph Flach & Sons, ltd.
Food Industries Ltd.
A. J. Gomiero Ltd. (V. Mane Fils S.A.)
A. W. Munns & Co., Ltd.
Natural & Synthetic Perfumery Essence Co.
Roure Bertrand Fils et Justin Dupont
Sōflor Ltd.
H. E. Stringer Ltd.
Alfred Paul White & Son
White, Tomkins & Courage Ltd.
Wilson & Mansfield Ltd.

OXIDES, IRON
(Brown & Black)
D. F. Anstead Ltd.
Barter Trading Corporation Ltd.
BASF United Kingdom Ltd.
Butterfield Laboratories Ltd.
Columbian International (Great Britain) Ltd.
H. J. Evans & Co., Ltd.
Golden Valley Colours Ltd.
W. Hawley & Son, Ltd.
Procter, Johnson & Co., Ltd.
C. E. Ramsden & Co., Ltd.
Shearman & Co., Ltd.

J. M. Steel & Co., Ltd.
Williams (Hounslow) Ltd.

OZOKERITE, WAX
Astor Boisselier & Lawrence Ltd.
British Wax Refining Co., Ltd.
Holroyd's Oil & Ceresine Co., Ltd.
H. Lattimer
Poth, Hille & Co., Ltd.
Renham & Romley Ltd.
Thew, Arnott & Co., Ltd.
Wilkins, Campbell & Co., Ltd.
Wynmouth Lehr & Fatoils Ltd.

PALMAROSA OIL
V. Berg & Sons, Ltd.
Blythe, Greene, Jourdain & Co., Ltd.
Bush Boake Allen Ltd., Perfumery Division
Charabot & Cie Ltd.
Antoine Chiris
F. D. Copeland & Sons, Ltd.
H. E. Daniel Ltd.
Fuerst Day Lawson Ltd.
Gale & Mount Ltd.
W. H. Hobbs & Co., Ltd.
A. W. Munns & Co., Ltd.
R. Sarant & Co., Ltd.
R. C. Treatt & Co. Ltd.
Wilson & Mansfield Ltd.
Chas. Zimmermann & Co., Ltd.

PALMITIC ACID
See suppliers of **Oleic** *and* **Stearic acids**

PARACYMENE
Hercules Powder Co., Ltd.
Kingsley & Keith (Chemicals) Ltd.
White Sea & Baltic Co., P. & I. Danischewsky Ltd.

PARAFFIN, LIQUID
See **Oils, mineral**

PARAFFIN WAX
See **Wax (paraffin)**

PATCHOULI OIL
V. Berg & Sons, Ltd.
Bertrand Freres Ltd.
Blyth, Greene, Jourdain & Co., Ltd.
Bush Boake Allen Ltd., Perfumery Division

Charabot & Cie Ltd.
Antoine Chiris Ltd.
F. D. Copeland & Sons, Ltd.
H. E. Daniel Ltd.
Felton Co. (Great Britain), Ltd.
Fuerst Day Lawson Ltd.
Gale & Mount Ltd.
A. J. Gomiero Ltd. (V. Mane Fils S.A.)
F. Gutkind & Co., Ltd.
A. G. Hersom
W. H. Hobbs & Co., Ltd.
John Kellys (London) Ltd.
Lautier Fils Ltd.
A. W. Munns & Co., Ltd.
Norda-Schimmel International Ltd.
Roure Bertrand Fils et Justin Dupont
P. Samuelson & Co., Ltd.
R. Sarant & Co., Ltd.
Sōflor Ltd.
H. E. Stringer Ltd.
R. C. Treatt & Co., Ltd.
Alfred Paul White & Son
Wilson & Mansfield Ltd.
Chas. Zimmermann & Co., Ltd.

PECTIN
T. M. Duché & Sons (U.K.), Ltd.
Esperis S.A.
F. Gutkind & Co., Ltd.
Kingsley & Keith (Chemicals) Ltd.
Union Glue & Gelatine Co., Ltd.

PEPPERMINT OIL
(ALL TYPES)
V. Berg & Sons, Ltd.
Bertrand Freres Ltd.
Blyth, Greene, Jourdain & Co., Ltd.
Bruce, Starke & Co., Ltd.
Bush Boake Allen Ltd., Perfumery Division
Charabot & Cie Ltd.
Cocker Chemical Co., Ltd.
F. D. Copeland & Sons, Ltd.
Courtin & Warner Ltd.
H. E. Daniel Ltd.
Dragoco (Gt. Britain) Ltd.
Felton Company (Great Britain) Ltd.
Food Industries Ltd.
Fuerst Day Lawson Ltd.

Gale & Mount Ltd.
A. J. Gomiero Ltd. (V. Mane Fils S.A.)
F. Gutkind & Co., Ltd.
T. Harrison & Co., Ltd.
A. G. Hersom
W. H. Hobbs & Co., Ltd.
Hollander Hyams Ltd.
Hollands Distillery (Essential Oils) Ltd.
International Flavours & Fragrances I.F.F. (Gt. Britain) Ltd.
John Kellys (London) Ltd.
Lautier Fils Ltd.
Lockwood, Magrath Pty. Ltd.
McVittie Anderson & Co., Ltd.
J. & G. Miller
A. W. Munns & Co., Ltd.
Norda-Schimmel International Ltd.
P. T. Petley & Co., Ltd.
Pigalle (International) Ltd.
William Ransom & Son, Ltd.
Roure Bertrand Fils et Justin Dupont
R. Sarant & Co., Ltd.
Sōflor Ltd.
Standard Synthetics Ltd.
Stevenson & Howell Ltd.
H. E. Stringer Ltd.
R. C. Treatt & Co., Ltd.
Alfred Paul White & Son
Wilson & Mansfield Ltd.
Chas. Zimmermann & Co., Ltd

PERFUMERY COMPOUNDS AND SPECIALITIES
See also **Aromatic chemicals** *and* **Essential oils**
Aromatica Ltd.
Atkins & Co.
Bertrand Freres Ltd.
Bruce, Starke & Co., Ltd.
Burmah Oil Trading Ltd. Lobitos Division
Bush Boake Allen Ltd., Perfumery Division
Charabot & Cie Ltd.
Antoine Chiris Ltd.
Courtin & Warner Ltd.
H. E. Daniel Ltd.
Dragoco (Gt. Britain) Ltd.
Dubuis & Rowsell Ltd.

Felton Company (Great Britain) Ltd.
Field & Co. (Aromatics), Ltd.
Firmenich Ltd.
Florasynth Ltd.
Gale & Mount Ltd.
Germstroyd Ltd.
Givaudan & Co., Ltd.
A. J. Gomiero Ltd. (V. Mane Fils S.A.)
R. W. Greeff & Co., Ltd.
Haarman & Reimer Ltd.
A. G. Hersom
W. H. Hobbs & Co., Ltd.
International Flavours & Fragrances I.F.F. (Great Britain) Ltd.
H. M. Langton & Co., Ltd.
Lautier Fils Ltd.
Leopold Laserson Ltd.
Lockwood Magrath Pty., Ltd.
Mallagh & Co.
May & Baker Ltd.
A. W. Munns & Co., Ltd.
'Naarden' (London) Ltd.
Natural & Synthetic Perfumery Essence Co.
Norda-Schimmel International Ltd.
P. T. Petley & Co., Ltd.
Pigalle (International) Ltd.
Proprietary Perfumes Ltd.
Roure Bertrand Fils et Justin Dupont
P. Samuelson & Co., Ltd.
R. Sarant & Co., Ltd.
Sōflor Ltd.
Standard Synthetics Ltd.
H. E. Stringer Ltd.
Supreme Mfg. Co., Ltd.
R. C. Treatt & Co., Ltd.
Ungerer & Co.
Alfred Paul White & Son
White Tomkins & Courage Ltd.
Wilson & Mansfield Ltd.
Chas. Zimmermann & Co., Ltd.

PEROXIDES
See also **Hydrogen peroxide**
The General Chemical Co., Ltd.
Hercules Powder Co., Ltd.
Imperial Chemical Industries Ltd.

Laporte Industries Ltd. (General Chemicals Division –Luton)
Novadel Ltd.
Sherman Chemicals Ltd.

PERSULPHATES
The General Chemical Co., Ltd.
Kingsley & Keith (Chemicals) Ltd.
Laporte Industries Ltd. (General Chemicals Division –Luton)
L. R. B. Pearce Ltd.
Sherman Chemicals Ltd.

PETITGRAIN
Bertrand Feres Ltd.
Blythe, Greene, Jourdain & Co., Ltd.
Bush Boake Allen Ltd., Perfumery Division
Charabot & Cie Ltd.
Antoine Chiris Ltd.
H. E. Daniel Ltd.
Dragoco (Gt. Britain) Ltd.
Food Industries Ltd.
Fuerst Day Lawson Ltd.
Gale & Mount Ltd.
A. J. Gomiero Ltd. (V. Mane Fils S.A.)
W. H. Hobbs & Co., Ltd.
Hollander Hyams Ltd.
Lautier Fils Ltd.
A. W. Munns & Co., Ltd.
Pigalle (International) Ltd.
Roure Bertrand Fils et Justin Dupont
P. Samuelson & Co., Ltd.
R. Sarant & Co., Ltd.
H. E. Stringer Ltd.
R. C. Treatt & Co., Ltd.
Alfred Paul White & Son
Wilson & Mansfield Ltd.
Chas. Zimmermann & Co., Ltd.

PETROLEUM JELLY
Alwitt Ltd.
Astor Boisselier & Lawrence Ltd.
Bartoline (Hull) Ltd.
Burmah Oil Trading Ltd. Lobitos Division
Holroyd's Oil & Ceresine Co., Ltd.
Meade-King Robinson & Co., Ltd.

L. R. B. Pearce Ltd.
Pharmaceutical Lanoline Co.
Printar Industries Ltd.
Purfinol Ltd.
Tar Residuals Ltd.
Wynmouth Lehr & Fatoils Ltd.
A. & M. Zimmermann

PHELLANDRENE
H. E. Daniel Ltd.
McVittie Anderson & Co., Ltd.
Standard Synthetics Ltd.
Wilson & Mansfield Ltd.

PHENOL
Coalite & Chemical Products
  Ltd.
The General Chemical Co.,
  Ltd.
James Greenshields & Co., Ltd.
Imperial Chemical Industries
  Ltd.
London Tar & Chemical Co.,
  Ltd.
Scottish Tar Distillers Ltd.
Tar Residuals Ltd.
The United Steel Companies
  Ltd.

PHENYLENEDIAMINE
(ORTHO, META AND
PARA)
Giba Clayton Ltd.
The General Chemical Co.,
  Ltd.
Hoechst Chemicals Ltd.
Imperial Chemical Industries
  Ltd.
Kingsley & Keith (Chemicals)
  Ltd.

PHENYLMERCURIC
SALTS
Berk Ltd.
Durham Raw Materials Ltd.
Imperial Chemical Industries
  Ltd.
Sherman Chemicals Ltd.
Tar Residuals Ltd.
Ward, Blenkinsop & Co., Ltd.

PINE TAR
Berk Ltd.
Bowring, Jones & Tidy Ltd.
A. V. Pound & Co., Ltd.
Tar Residuals Ltd.
Westwood Macneill & Co., Ltd.
White Sea & Baltic Co.,
  P. & I. Danischewsky Ltd.
Wynmouth Lehr & Fatoils Ltd.

POLYETHYLENE
GLYCOLS
Glovers (Chemicals) Ltd.
Geo. T. Gurr Ltd.
Hoechst Chemicals Ltd.
Honeywill & Stein Ltd.
Imperial Chemical Industries
  Ltd.
Jacobson Van Den Berg & Co.
  (U.K.), Ltd.
Kingsley & Keith (Chemicals)
  Ltd.
Lankro Chemicals Ltd.
E. J. R. Lovelock
A. Revai & Co. (Chemicals),
  Ltd.
Shell Chemical U.K. Ltd.
Tar Residuals Ltd.
Union Carbide Ltd. (Chemicals
  Division)

POLYETHYLENE
GLYCOL ESTERS
See under **Emulsifying
agents**

POLYVINYL
COMPOUNDS
Fine Dyestuffs & Chemicals
  Ltd.
Hoechst Chemicals Ltd.
Honeywill & Stein Ltd.
Imperial Chemical Industries
  Ltd.
National Adhesives Ltd.
Scott Bader & Co., Ltd.
Shawinigan Ltd.

POLYVINYL
PYROLLIDONE
BASF United Kingdom Ltd.
Victor Blagden & Co., Ltd.
British Oxygen Co., Ltd.
Fine Dyestuffs & Chemicals
  Ltd.

POTASH
See **Potassium carbonate**

POTASH, CAUSTIC
See **Potassium hydroxide**

POTASSIUM
BICARBONATE
Berk Ltd.
The General Chemical Co.,
  Ltd.
Thomas Morson & Son, Ltd.
Tar Residuals Ltd.

POTASSIUM
CARBONATE
Berk Ltd.
H. J. Evans & Co., Ltd.
The General Chemical Co.,
  Ltd.
Millwards Merchandise Ltd.
Thomas Morson & Son, Ltd.
Tar Residuals Ltd.

POTASSIUM
HYDROXIDE
Berk Ltd.
East Lancashire Chemical Co.,
  Ltd.
The General Chemical Co.,
  Ltd.
Imperial Chemical Industries
  Ltd.
Kingsley & Keith (Chemicals)
  Ltd.
May & Baker Ltd.
Thomas Morson & Son, Ltd.
L. E. Pritchitt & Co., Ltd.
Sherman Chemicals Ltd.
Tar Residuals Ltd.

POTASSIUM NITRATE
Berk Ltd.
Courtin & Warner Ltd.
The General Chemical Co.,
  Ltd.
James Greenshields & Co., Ltd.
Imperial Chemical Industries
  Ltd.
Thomas Morson & Son, Ltd.
L. E. Pritchitt & Co., Ltd.
Sherman Chemicals Ltd.
Tar Residuals Ltd.

POTASSIUM
PERMANGANATE
Courtin & Warner Ltd.
The General Chemical Co.,
  Ltd.
Millwards Merchandise Ltd.
Thomas Morson & Son, Ltd.
Sherman Chemicals Ltd.
Tar Residuals Ltd.
A. & M. Zimmermann

POTASH SALTS
(VARIOUS)
A.B.M. Industrial Products
  Ltd.
The General Chemical Co.,
  Ltd.
Hardman & Holden Ltd.
Millwards Merchandise Ltd.

Tar Residuals Ltd.

POT POURRI MATERIALS
Atkins & Co.
Bertrand Freres Ltd.
Dragoco (Gt. Britain) Ltd.
Joseph Flach & Sons, Ltd.

POWDER BRUSHES
Percy P. Baker Ltd.
Cope Allman Packaging
Geo. T. Gurr Ltd.
A. V. Pound & Co., Ltd.
Team Valley Brush Co., Ltd.

POWDER PUFFS
Caressa Ltd.
L. Kahn Mfg. Co., Ltd.
Lambournes (B'ham) Ltd.
A. J. Siris Products Ltd.
Solport Bros. Ltd

PRESERVATIVES (for Cosmetics)
See also **Antioxidants**
Bush Boake Allen Ltd.,
  Perfumery Division
Distillers Chemicals & Plastics
  Ltd.
Fine Dyestuffs & Chemicals
  Ltd.
Imperial Chemical Industries
  Ltd.
Industrial Solvents Division
Pfizer Ltd.
Ward, Blenkinsop & Co., Ltd.

PROPYLENE GLYCOL
BASF United Kingdom Ltd.
The General Chemical Co.,
  Ltd.
R. W. Greeff & Co., Ltd.
Imperial Chemical Industries
  Ltd.
Kingsley & Keith (Chemicals)
  Ltd.
Shell Chemical U.K. Ltd.
Standard Synthetics Ltd.
Union Carbide Ltd. (Chemicals
  Division)

PUMICE
Richard Baker & Co., Ltd.
M. J. Fecher Ltd.
Jessop & Co.
Procter, Johnson & Co., Ltd.
Solport Bros. Ltd.
Thew, Arnott & Co., Ltd.
A. & M. Zimmermann

PYRIDINE
Ango-Scottish Chemical Co.,
  Ltd.
Victor Blagden & Co., Ltd.
The General Chemical Co.,
  Ltd.
James Greenshields & Co., Ltd.
Kingsley & Keith (Chemicals)
  Ltd.
Lancashire Tar Distillers Ltd.
Tar Residuals Ltd.
Westwood Macneill & Co., Ltd.

QUASSIA CHIPS AND EXTRACTS
V. Berg & Sons, Ltd.
Bush Boake Allen Ltd.,
  Perfumery Division
H. E. Daniel Ltd.
Joseph Flach & Sons, Ltd.
John Kellys (London) Ltd.
Wm. Ransom & Son, Ltd.
White, Tompkins & Courage
  Ltd.

QUATERNARY AMMONIUM COMPOUNDS
Alwitt Ltd.
Berk Ltd.
Victor Blagden & Co., Ltd.
British Hydrological
  Corporation
Ciba Clayton Ltd.
Cyclo Chemicals Ltd.
Dutton & Reinisch Ltd.
Fine Dyestuffs & Chemicals
  Ltd.
The General Chemical Co.,
  Ltd.
Glovers (Chemicals) Ltd.
Guest Industrials Ltd.
Hoechst Chemicals Ltd.
Imperial Chemical Industries
  Ltd.
Keegan Dyestuffs & Chemicals
  Ltd.
Lennig Chemicals Ltd.
Novadel Ltd.
Printar Industries Ltd.
Ronsheim & Moore Ltd.
J. M. Steel & Co., Ltd.
J. C. Thompson & Co. (Duron),
  Ltd.
Ward, Blenkinsop & Co., Ltd.

QUINCE SEEDS
Joseph Flach & Sons, Ltd.

H. Frischmann
F. Gutkind & Co., Ltd.
John Kellys (London) Ltd.
H. Lattimer

QUININE SALTS
Victor Blagden & Co., Ltd.
Courtin & Warner Ltd.
Chas. Zimmermann & Co.,
  Ltd.

RECTIFIED SPIRIT
See **Alcohol (S.V.R.)**

RED OCHRE
D. F. Anstead Ltd.
Butterfield Laboratories Ltd.
Columbian International (Gt.
  Britain) Ltd.
H. J. Evans & Co., Ltd.
Golden Valley Colours Ltd.
W. Hawley & Son, Ltd.

RESINS, OLEO-RESINS and BALSAMS
Bush Boake Allen Ltd.,
  Perfumery Division
Charabot & Cie Ltd.
Antoine Chiris Ltd.
Courtin & Warner Ltd.
H. E. Daniel Ltd.
Dragoco (Gt. Britain) Ltd.
Florasynth Ltd.
Food Industries Ltd.
H. Frischmann
Fuerst Day Lawson Ltd.
Geigy (U.K.) Ltd.
Natural & Synthetic Perfumery
  Essence Co.
Pigalle (International) Ltd.
Wm. Ransom & Son, Ltd.
H. E. Stringer Ltd.
Alfred Paul White & Son
White, Tomkins & Courage
  Ltd.
Wilson & Mansfield Ltd.

RESINS, SYNTHETIC
Barter Trading Corporation
  Ltd.
Bartoline (Hull) Ltd.
Ciba Clayton Ltd.
Corn Products (Sales) Ltd.
Cornelius Chemical Co., Ltd.
Elga Products Ltd.
Florasynth Ltd.
Geigy (U.K.) Ltd.
Hercules Powder Co. Ltd.
Hoechst Chemicals Ltd.

Howards of Ilford Ltd.
Imperial Chemical Industries Ltd.
Scott, Bader & Co., Ltd.
Shell Chemical U.K. Ltd.
Standard Synthetics Ltd.
H. E. Stringer Ltd.
Tar Residuals Ltd.
United Coke & Chemicals Co., Ltd.
Victor Wolf Ltd.

RIBBONS (Plain and Fancy)
Charles Clay & Sons Ltd.
John Maclennan (Textiles & Insulating Materials) Ltd.
Porth Textiles Ltd.
Tyruplex Ltd.

RICE STARCH
V. Berg & Sons, Ltd.
Laing-National Ltd.

ROSE (Concrete, Absolute, etc.)
Bertrand Freres Ltd.
Bush Boake Allen Ltd., Perfumery Division
Charabot & Cie Ltd.
Antoine Chiris Ltd.
F. D. Copeland & Sons, Ltd.
Jean A. du Crocq Jr. N.V.
Dragoco (Gt. Britain) Ltd.
W. H. Hobbs & Co. Ltd.
Lautier Fils Ltd.
A. W. Munns & Co., Ltd.
Natural & Synthetic Perfumery Essence Co., Ltd.
Norda-Schimmel International Ltd.
P. T. Petley & Co., Ltd.
Pigalle (International) Ltd.
Roure Bertrand Fils et Justin Dupont
R. Sarant & Co., Ltd.
Sōflor Ltd.
H. E. Stringer Ltd.
Alfred Paul White & Son
Wilson & Mansfield Ltd.

ROSE OTTO
Bertrand Freres Ltd.
Bush Boake Allen Ltd., Perfumery Division
Charabot & Cie Ltd.
Antoine Chiris Ltd.
F. D. Copeland & Sons, Ltd.
Dragoco (Gt. Britain) Ltd.

Dubuis & Rowsell Ltd.
Fuerst Day Lawson Ltd.
W. H. Hobbs & Co., Ltd.
H. M. Langton & Co., Ltd.
Lautier Fils Ltd.
A. W. Munns & Co., Ltd.
Norda-Schimmel International Ltd.
Roure Bertrand Fils et Justin Dupont
R. Sarant & Co., Ltd.
Sōflor Ltd.
R. C. Treatt & Co., Ltd.
Alfred Paul White & Son
Wilson & Mansfield Ltd.

ROSEMARY
Bertrand Freres Ltd.
Bush Boake Allen Ltd., Perfumery Division
Charabot & Cie Ltd.
Antoine Chiris Ltd.
F. D. Copeland & Sons, Ltd.
Courtin & Warner Ltd.
H. E. Daniel Ltd.
Joseph Flach & Sons, Ltd.
Food Industries Ltd.
Fuerst Day Lawson Ltd.
Gale & Mount Ltd.
A. J. Gomiero Ltd. (V. Mane Fils S.A.)
F. Gutkind & Co., Ltd.
A. G. Hersom
M. Agusti Hidalgo (London) Ltd.
W. H. Hobbs & Co., Ltd.
Lautier Fils Ltd.
A. W. Munns & Co., Ltd.
Norda-Schimmel International Ltd.
Pigalle (International) Ltd.
Roure Bertrand Fils et Justin Dupont
P. Samuelson & Co., Ltd.
R. Sarant & Co., Ltd.
Standard Synthetics Ltd.
H. E. Stringer Ltd.
R. C. Treatt & Co., Ltd.
Alfred Paul White & Son
Wilson & Mansfield Ltd.
Chas. Zimmermann & Co.., Ltd.

ROSIN
Berk Ltd.
Bowring, Jones & Tidy Ltd.
British Celanese Ltd.
H. E. Daniel Ltd.

F. Gutkind & Co., Ltd.
Hercules Powder Co. Ltd.
Langley-Smith & Co., Ltd.
Meade-King, Robinson & Co., Ltd.
A. V. Pound & Co., Ltd.
Shearman & Co., Ltd.
Smith & Forrest (Oils) Ltd.
Tar Residuals Ltd.
White Sea & Baltic Co., P. & I. Danischewsky Ltd.
Thew, Arnott & Co., Ltd.
Wynmouth Lehr & Fatoils Ltd.

ROSIN, Liquid
Berk Ltd.
Bowring, Jones & Tidy Ltd.
E. J. R. Lovelock
Meade-King, Robinson & Co., Ltd.
A. V. Pound & Co., Ltd.
Shearman & Co. Ltd.
Tar Residuals Ltd.
White Sea & Baltic Co., P. & I. Danischewsky Ltd.
Wynmouth Lehr & Fatoils Ltd.

SACCHARIN
Food Industries Ltd.
Kingsley & Keith (Chemicals) Ltd.

SACHETS, PERFUMERY
Alcan Foils Ltd.
Atkins & Company
Convertex Machinery Ltd.
L. Kahn Mfg. Co., Ltd.
Metal Box Co., Ltd.
John Tye & Son, Ltd.

SANDALWOOD OIL (EAST INDIAN)
V. Berg & Sons, Ltd.
Blyth, Greene, Jourdain & Co., Ltd.
Bush Boake Allen Ltd., Perfumery Division
Charabot & Cie Ltd.
F. D. Copeland & Sons, Ltd.
H. E. Daniel Ltd.
Dragoco (Gt. Britain) Ltd.
Felton Co. (Gt. Britain), Ltd.
Fuerst Day Lawson Ltd.
Gale & Mount Ltd.
A. J. Gomiero Ltd. (V. Mane Fils S.A.)
F. Gutkind & Co., Ltd.
A. G. Hersom
W. H. Hobbs & Co.

193

Hollander Hyams Ltd.
Lautier Fils Ltd.
McVittie Anderson & Co., Ltd.
A. W. Munns & Co., Ltd.
Roure Bertrand Fils et Justin
Dupont
R. Sarant & Co., Ltd.
Sõflor Ltd.
Trade Agent for Mysore in
London.
R. C. Treatt & Co., Ltd.
Alfred Paul White & Son
Wilson & Mansfield Ltd.
Chas. Zimmermann & Co.,
Ltd.

SANDALWOOD OIL (W. AUSTRALIAN)
Bush Boake Allen Ltd.,
Perfumery Division
H. E. Daniel Ltd.
Fuerst Day Lawson Ltd.
Gale & Mount Ltd.
A. G. Hersom
W. H. Hobbs & Co. Ltd.
Lautier Fils Ltd.
McVittie Anderson & Co., Ltd.
Sõflor Ltd.

SAPONIN
Bush Boake Allen Ltd.,
Perfumery Division
Food Industries Ltd.
Kingsley & Keith (Chemicals)
Ltd.

SASSAFRASS OIL
V. Berg & Sons, Ltd.
Bertrand Freres Ltd.
Blyth, Greene, Jourdain & Co.,
Ltd.
Bush Boake Allen Ltd.,
Perfumery Division
Charabot & Cie Ltd.
Courtin & Warner Ltd.
H. E. Daniel Ltd.
Joseph Flach & Sons, Ltd.
Food Industries Ltd.
Fuerst Day Lawson Ltd.
Gale & Mount Ltd.
W. H. Hobbs & Co., Ltd.
Hollander Hyams Ltd.
A. W. Munns & Co., Ltd.
R. Sarant & Co., Ltd.
R. C. Treatt & Co., Ltd.
Wilson & Mansfield Ltd.
Chas. Zimmermann & Co.,
Ltd.

SEQUESTERING AGENTS
See **Ethylene diamine tetra
acetic acid**

SHAMPOO BASES
See under **Soaps,
soft and powder;** also
under **Sulphonated
alcohols** etc.

SHELLAC
V. Berg & Sons, Ltd.
H. E. Daniel Ltd.
M. Hamburger & Sons, Ltd.
Honeywill & Steiner Ltd.
H. Lattimer
Shearman & Co., Ltd.
Thew, Arnott & Co., Ltd.
Thews Ltd.

SIENNA (BURNT AND RAW)
D. F. Anstead Ltd.
Golden Valley Colours Ltd.
W. Hawley & Son, Ltd.
Procter, Johnson & Co., Ltd.
Shearman & Co., Ltd.
Williams (Hounslow) Ltd.

SIENNAS
See **Oxides, iron**

SILICA
Richard Baker & Co., Ltd.
Cornwall Mills Ltd.
A. Elder Reed & Co., Ltd.
H. J. Evans & Co., Ltd.
Hardman & Holden Ltd.
Scientific Glass-Blowing Co.
Shearman & Co., Ltd.
Thermal Syndicate Ltd.

SILICA (GROUND)
Richard Baker & Co., Ltd.
Bush Beach & Segner Bayley
Ltd.
Cornwall Mills Ltd.
H. J. Evans & Co., Ltd.
W. Hawley & Son, Ltd.
C. E. Ramsden & Co., Ltd.

SILICA, AMORPHOUS
Bush, Beach & Segner Bayley
Ltd.
Joseph Crosfield & Sons, Ltd.
Peter Spence & Sons, Ltd.

SILICA, DIATOMACEOUS
Johns-Manville (Gt. Britain)
Ltd.
Tar Residuals Ltd.

SILICATE OF SODA
See **Sodium silicate**

SILICONES
Jacobson Van Der Berg & Co.
(U.K.), Ltd.
Midland Silicones Ltd.
J. C. Thompson & Co. (Duron),
Ltd.

SODA ASH (Crude Sodium Carbonate)
Imperial Chemical Industries
Ltd.

SODA-LIME
General Chemical Co., Ltd.

SODIUM ALGINATE
See under **Alginates**

SODIUM BICARBONATE
Frederick Allen & Sons
(Chemicals), Ltd.
Food Industries Ltd.
The General Chemical Co.,
Ltd.
Howards of Ilford Ltd.
Imperial Chemical Industries
Ltd.
Jessop & Co.
Laporte Industries Ltd.
(Organics & Pigments
Division–Ilford)
Millwards Merchandise Ltd.
Thomas Morson & Son, Ltd.

SODIUM BICHROMATE
Associated Chemical
Companies (Mfg.) Ltd.
The General Chemical Co.,
Ltd.
Keegan Dyestuffs & Chemicals
Ltd.
Millwards Merchandise Ltd.
Thomas Morson & Son, Ltd.
Tar Residuals Ltd.

SODIUM CARBONATE (Pure)
The General Chemical Co.,
Ltd.
Howards of Ilford Ltd.
Imperial Chemical Industries
Ltd.
Laporte Industries Ltd.
(Organics & Pigments
Division–Ilford)
Millwards Merchandise Ltd.
Thomas Morson & Son, Ltd.
Sherman Chemicals Ltd.

SODIUM CARBONATE MONOHYDRATE
The General Chemical Co., Ltd.
Howards of Ilford Ltd.
Imperial Chemical Industries Ltd.
Kingsley & Keith (Chemicals) Ltd.

SODIUM CHLORATE
Berk Ltd.
Victor Blagden & Co., Ltd.
British Anhydrous Ammonia Co., Ltd.
The General Chemical Co., Ltd.
R. W. Greeff & Co., Ltd.
Guest Industrials Ltd.
Harrison Clark Ltd.
Millwards Merchandise Ltd.
Thomas Morson & Son, Ltd.
L. R. B. Pearce Ltd.
J. M. Steel & Co., Ltd.
Synthite Ltd.
Tar Residuals Ltd.

SODIUM CHLORIDE
Barter Trading Corporation Ltd.
Berk Ltd.
The General Chemical Co., Ltd.
Howards of Ilford Ltd.
Imperial Chemical Industries Ltd.
May & Baker Ltd.
Millwards Merchandise Ltd.
Thomas Morson & Son, ltd.

SODIUM HYDROSULPHITE
Associated Chemical Companies (Mfg.) Ltd.
Ciba Clayton Ltd.
Hardman & Holden Ltd.
Millwards Merchandise Ltd.
Tar Residuals Ltd.

SODIUM HYDROXIDE
Frederick Allen & Sons (Chemicals), Ltd.
Barter Trading Corporation Ltd.
Berk Ltd.
East Lancashire Chemical Co., Ltd.
The General Chemical Co., Ltd.

Imperial Chemical Industries Ltd.
Jessop & Co.
May & Baker Ltd.
Millwards Merchandise Ltd.
Thomas Morson & Son, Ltd.
L. R. B. Pearce Ltd.
L. E. Pritchitt & Co., Ltd.
Sherman Chemicals Ltd.
Staveley Chemicals Ltd.

SODIUM LAURYL SULPHATE
See under **Alcohols, sulphated fatty**

SODIUM METABORATE
Borax Consolidated Ltd.
The General Chemical Co., Ltd.

SODIUM META-PHOSPHATE
The General Chemical Co., Ltd.

SODIUM METASILICATE
Alcock (Peroxide) Ltd.
Berk Ltd.
Brown & Forth Ltd.
Joseph Crosfield & Sons, Ltd.
The General Chemical Co., Ltd.
Imperial Chemical Industries Ltd.
Laporte Industries Ltd. (General Chemicals Division)
Millwards Merchandise Ltd.

SODIUM PERBORATE
Brown & Forth Ltd.
The General Chemical Co., Ltd.
Imperial Chemical Industries Ltd.
Laporte Industries Ltd. (General Chemicals Division–Luton)
Millwards Merchandise Ltd.

SODIUM PERCARBONATE
Brown & Forth Ltd.
Imperial Chemical Industries Ltd.
The General Chemical Co., Ltd.
Laporte Industries Ltd. (General Chemicals

Division–Luton)
Millwards Merchandise Ltd.

SODIUM PEROXIDE
The General Chemical Co., Ltd.
Imperial Chemical Industries Ltd.
Millwards Merchandise Ltd.

SODIUM PHOSPHATE (DIBASIC)
The General Chemical Co., Ltd.
Millwards Merchandise Ltd.
Thomas Morson & Son, Ltd.

SODIUM PHOSPHATE (TRIBASIC)
The General Chemical Co., Ltd.
Millwards Merchandise Ltd.
Thomas Morson & Son, Ltd.
Tar Residuals Ltd.

SODIUM PYROPHOSPHATE
The General Chemical Co., Ltd.

SODIUM SESQUICARBONATE
The General Chemical Co., Ltd.
Imperial Chemical Industries Ltd.
Millwards Merchandise Ltd.

SODIUM SILICATE
Joseph Crosfield & Sons, Ltd.
H. J. Evans & Co., Ltd.
The General Chemical Co., Ltd.
Imperial Chemical Industries Ltd.
Millwards Merchandise Ltd.
Tar Residuals Ltd.

SODIUM SULPHATE (GLAUBER'S SALT)
Associated Chemical Companies (Mfg.) Ltd.
Berk Ltd.
W. Blythe & Co., Ltd.
British Anhydrous Ammonia Co., Ltd.
British Celanese Ltd.
H. J. Evans & Co., Ltd.
The General Chemical Co., Ltd.

Harris Hart & Co., Ltd
Howards of Ilford Ltd.
Imperial Chemical Industries
  Ltd.
Laporte Industries Ltd.
  (Organics & Pigments
  Division–Ilford)
Millwards Merchandise Ltd.
Thomas Morson & Son, Ltd.
J. M. Steel & Co., Ltd.
Tar Residuals Ltd.
Westwood Macneill & Co., Ltd.

SODIUM SULPHIDE (PURE)
The General Chemical Co.,
  Ltd.
Imperial Chemical Industries
  Ltd.
Millwards Merchandise Ltd.
Thomas Morson & Son, Ltd.
Sherman Chemicals Ltd.
Tar Residuals Ltd.

SODIUM SULPHITES
A.B.M. Industrial Products
  Ltd.
Associated Chemical
  Companies (Mfg.) Ltd.
Berk Ltd.
W. Blythe & Co., Ltd.
The General Chemical Co.,
  Ltd.
James Greenshields & Co., Ltd.
Imperial Chemical Industries
  Ltd.
L. R. B. Pearce Ltd.
Millwards Merchandise Ltd.

SODIUM THIOSULPHATE
W. Blythe & Co., Ltd.
The General Chemical Co.,
  Ltd.
Imperial Chemical Industries
  Ltd.
Millwards Merchandise Ltd.
Thomas Morson & Son, Ltd.

SOLVENTS
See also under **Alcohol** *and
other specific headings*
Alwitt Ltd.
BSAF United Kingdom Ltd.
British Celanese Ltd.
The General Chemical Co.,
  Ltd.
Hoechst Chemicals Ltd.
Honeywill & Stein Ltd

Howards of Ilford Ltd.
Imperial Chemical Industries
  Ltd.
Kingsley & Keith (Chemicals)
  Ltd.
Lancashire Tar Distillers Ltd.
Laporte Industries Ltd.
  (Organics & Pigments
  Division–Ilford)
May & Baker Ltd.
Meade-King, Robinson & Co.,
  Ltd.
Methylating Co., Ltd.
Millwards Merchandise Ltd.
A. Revai & Co. (Chemicals),
  Ltd.
Shell Chemicals U.K. Ltd.
Sherman Chemicals Ltd.
Tar Residuals Ltd.
Union Carbide Ltd. (Chemicals
  Division)

SORBIC ACID
A.B.M. Industrial Products
  Ltd.
Victor Blagden & Co., Ltd.
Distillers Chemicals & Plastics
  Ltd.
Hoechst Chemicals Ltd.

SORBITOL
Berk Ltd.
Bio-Cosmetic Research
  Laboratories
Howards of Ilford Ltd.
Laporte Industries Ltd.
  (Organics & Pigments
  Division–Ilford)
Kingsley & Keith (Chemicals)
  Ltd.
L. R. B. Pearce Ltd.

SORBITOL DERIVATIVES
Berk Ltd.
Victor Blagden & Co., Ltd.
Rex Campbell & Co., Ltd.
Croda Ltd.
Howards of Ilford Ltd.
Leek Chemicals ltd.

SPERMACETI
Bio-Cosmetic Research
  Laboratories
Cyclo Chemicals Ltd.
H. E. Daniel Ltd.
Joseph Flach & Sons, Ltd.
Highgate & Job Ltd.

Holroyd's Oil & Ceresine Co.,
  Ltd.
H. Lattimer
E. J. R. Lovelock
Millwards Merchandise Ltd.
W. C. Smithie & Co., Ltd.
Thew, Arnott & Co., Ltd.
Velho Blackstock & Co., Ltd.
Wynmouth Lehr & Fatoils Ltd.

SPIKE OIL
Bertrand Freres Ltd.
Bruce, Starke & Co., Ltd.
Charabot & Cie Ltd.
Antoine Chiris Ltd.
F. D. Copeland & Sons, Ltd.
H. E. Daniel Ltd.
Dragoco (Gt. Britain) Ltd.
Gale & Mount Ltd.
A. J. Gomiero Ltd. (V. Mane
  Fils S.A.)
F. Gutkind & Co., Ltd.
A. G. Hersom
W. H. Hobbs & Co., Ltd.
Lautier Fils Ltd.
Mallagh & Co.
A. W. Munns & Co., Ltd.
Norda-Schimmel International
  Ltd.
Roure Bertrand Fils et Justin
  Dupont
P. Samuelson & Co., Ltd.
R. Sarant & Co., Ltd.
Standard Synthetics Ltd.
R. C. Treatt & Co., Ltd.
Alfred Paul White & Son.
Wilson & Mansfield Ltd.
Chas. Zimmermann & Co.,
  Ltd.

SPIRITS OF WINE
See **Alcohol (S.V.R.)**

SPIRITS, METHYLATED
See **Alcohol (I.M.S.)**

STARCHES (ALL TYPES)
Bruce, Stark & Co., Ltd.
Laing-National Ltd.
H. Lattimer
Millwards Merchandise Ltd.
Harry B. Wood Ltd.

STEAM TRAPS
Lancaster & Tonge Ltd.
Royles Ltd.

STEARAMIDE
See under **Amides, fatty**

196

STEARATES

Berk Ltd.
J. Bibby & Sons, Ltd.
Bush Boake Allen Ltd.,
　Perfumery Division
Rex Campbell & Co., Ltd.
Dunn Bros. Manchester Ltd.
Durham Raw Materials Ltd.
Food Industries Ltd.
The General Chemical Co.,
　Ltd.
M. Hamburger & Sons, Ltd.
Hardman & Holden Ltd.
Imperial Chemical Industries
　Ltd.
Keegan Dyestuffs & Chemicals
　Ltd.
H. Lattimer
Leek Chemicals Ltd.
E. J. R. Lovelock
Sandeman Bros., Ltd.
J. C. Thompson & Co. (Duron),
　Ltd.
Union Carbide Ltd.

STEARIC ACID

Armour Hess Chemicals Ltd.
S. Bramwell & Co., Ltd.
Rex Campbell & Co., Ltd.
Croda Ltd.
Cyclo Chemicals Ltd.
Durham Raw Materials Ltd.
Edipro Ltd.
The General Chemical Co.,
　Ltd.
M. Hamburger & Sons, Ltd.
Kingsley & Keith (Chemicals)
　Ltd.
E. J. R. Lovelock
Meade-King, Robinson & Co.,
　Ltd.
Millwards Merchandise Ltd.
Thomas Morson & Son, Ltd.
Price's (Bromborough) Ltd.
Universal Oil Co., Ltd.
Velho Blackstock & Co., Ltd.
John Waddington & Sons, Ltd.
Victor Wolf Ltd.
Wynmouth Lehr & Fatoils Ltd.

STEARINES

Armour Hess Chemicals Ltd.
S. Bramwell & Co., Ltd.
Food Industries Ltd.
M. Hamburger & Sons, Ltd.
E. J. R. Lovelock
Meade-King, Robinson & Co.,
　Ltd.

Price's (Bromborough) Ltd.
Thew, Arnott & Co., Ltd.
J. C. Thompson & Co. (Duron),
　Ltd.
Universal Oil Co., Ltd.
Velho Blackstock & Co., Ltd.
Wynmouth Lehr & Fatoils Ltd.

STEARYL ALCOHOL

Bio-Cosmetic Research
　Laboratories
Rex Campbell & Co., Ltd.
Croda Ltd.
Cyclo Chemicals Ltd.
The General Chemical Co.,
　Ltd.
R. W. Greeff & Co., Ltd.
Keegan Dyestuffs & Chemicals
　Ltd.
Kingsley & Keith (Chemicals)
　Ltd.
E. J. R. Lovelock
Marchon Products Ltd.
Price's (Bromborough) Ltd.
Ronsheim & Moore Ltd.
Sipon Products Ltd.

STILLS, WATER

Adelphi Mfg. Co., Ltd.
Apex Construction Ltd.
Baird & Tatlock Ltd.
Brown & Son (Alembic Works),
　Ltd.
George Cohen, Sons & Co.,
　Ltd.
John Dore & Co., Ltd.
Fisons Scientific Apparatus
　Ltd.
A. Gallenkamp & Co., Ltd.
Hospital & Laboratory
　Supplies Ltd.
Manesty Machines Ltd.
Townson & Mercer Ltd.

STRONTIUM SULPHIDE

Sherman Chemicals Ltd.

SULPHOCARBOLATES

Thomas Morson & Son, Ltd.

SULPHO-SUCCINATE COMPOUNDS

A. B. M. Industrial Products
　Ltd.
Victor Blagden & Co., Ltd.
Dutton & Reinisch Ltd.
Glovers (Chemicals) Ltd.
Kingsley & Keith (Chemicals)
　Ltd.

SULPHUR

BASF United Kindom Ltd.
Berk Ltd.
W. Blythe & Co., Ltd.
H. J. Evans & Co., Ltd.
The General Chemical Co.,
　Ltd.
Jessop & Co.
Shell Chemical U.K. Ltd.

SULPHUR, COLLOIDAL

BASF United Kingdom Ltd.
Bio-Cosmetic Research
　Laboratories
Keegan Dyestuffs & Chemicals
　Ltd.
Kingsley & Keith (Chemicals)
　Ltd.
Sherman Chemicals Ltd.

SUN SCREENING AGENTS

D. F. Anstead Ltd.
Bio-Cosmetic Research
　Laboratories
Bush Boake Allen Ltd.,
　Perfumery Division
Dragoco (Gt. Britain) Ltd.
Felton Co. (Gt. Britain), Ltd.
Fine Dyestuffs & Chemicals
　Ltd.
Firmenich Ltd.
Givaudan Co., Ltd.
Nipa Laboratories Ltd.
Ward, Blenkinsop & Co., Ltd.

TALC

D. F. Anstead Ltd.
Richard Baker & Co., Ltd.
Berk Ltd.
Blackwell's Metallurgical
　Works Ltd.
Durham Raw Materials Ltd.
H. J. Evans & Co., Ltd.
Golden Valley Colours Ltd.
W. Harrison & Co., Ltd.
Jessop & Co.
A. Levermore & Co., Ltd.
Procter, Johnson & Co., Ltd.
Shearman & Co., Ltd.
A. J. Siris Products Ltd.
Taylor Bros. & Cox Ltd.
Thew, Arnott & Co., Ltd.
Zach Cartwright Ltd.
A. & M. Zimmermann

TALLOW

Henry Barlow & Sons (Oils),
　Ltd.

S. Bramwell & Co., Ltd.
M. Hamburger & Sons, Ltd.
Holroyd's Oil & Ceresine Co., Ltd.
Langley-Smith & Co., Ltd.
Meade-King Robinson & Co., Ltd.
Millwards Merchandise Ltd.
Thew, Arnott & Co., Ltd.
Velho, Blackstock & Co., Ltd.
John Waddington & Sons, Ltd.
Wynmouth Lehr & Fatoils Ltd.

TAR PRODUCTS
See also **Acid (carbolic)**
Anglo-Scottish Chemical Co., Ltd.
Coalite & Chemical Products Ltd.
James Greenshields & Co., Ltd.
Lancashire Tar Distillers Ltd.
Scottish Tar Distillers Ltd.
Tar Residuals Ltd.
United Coke & Chemicals Co., Ltd.
The United Steel Companies Ltd.
Westwood Macneill & Co., Ltd.
The White Sea & Baltic Co., P. & I. Danischewsky Ltd.

TEREBENE
Bartoline (Hull) Ltd.
Bowring, Jones & Tidy Ltd.
Bush Boake Allen Ltd., Perfumery Division
Rex Campbell & Co., Ltd.

TERPINEOL
See also under **Aromatic Chemicals**
V. Berg & Sons, Ltd.
Bertrand Freres Ltd.
Bush Boake Allen Ltd., Perfumery Division
Rex Campbell & Co., Ltd.
Cocker Chemical Co., Ltd.
H. E. Daniel Ltd.
Fuerst Day Lawson Ltd.
Hercules Powder Co., Ltd.
May & Baker Ltd.
A. W. Munns & Co., Ltd.
Standard Synthetics Ltd.
Wilson & Mansfield Ltd.
Wynmouth Lehr & Fatoils Ltd.

TERPINOLENE
Bertrand Freres Ltd.
Bruce Starke & Co., Ltd.

Bush Boake Allen Ltd., Perfumery Division
Rex Campbell & Co., Ltd.
Cocker Chemical Co., Ltd.
H. E. Daniel Ltd.
Honeywill & Stein Ltd.
Standard Synthetics Ltd.
Wilson & Mansfield Ltd.
Wynmouth Lehr & Fatoils Ltd.

THIOUREA
Alwitt Ltd.
Victor Blagden & Co. Ltd.
The General Chemical Co., Ltd.
Hardman & Holden Ltd.
Kingsley & Keith (Chemicals) Ltd.
A. Revai & Co. (Chemicals), Ltd.

THYME
Bertrand Freres
Bush Boake Allen Ltd., Perfumery Division
Charabot & Cie Ltd.
H. E. Daniel Ltd.
Joseph Flach & Sons, Ltd.
Food Industries Ltd.
Fuerst Day Lawson Ltd.
Gale & Mount Ltd.
A. J. Gomiero Ltd. (V. Mane Fils S.A.).
F. Gutkind & Co., Ltd.
W. H. Hobbs & Co., Ltd.
John Kellys (London) Ltd.
Lautier Fils Ltd.
McVittie Anderson & Co., Ltd.
A. W. Munns & Co., Ltd.
Norda-Schimmel International Ltd.
Pigalle (International) Ltd.
Roure Bertrand Fils et Justin Dupont
H. Rubeck Ltd.
Standard Synthetics Ltd.
R. C. Treatt & Co., Ltd.
Alfred Paul White & Son
Wilson & Mansfield Ltd.
Chas. Zimmermann & Co. Ltd.

THYMOL
Bertrand Freres Ltd.
Rex Campbell & Co., Ltd.
Courtin & Warner Ltd.
H. E. Daniel Ltd.
The General Chemical Co., Ltd.

Howards of Ilford Ltd.
Laporte Industries Ltd. (Organics & Pigments Division–Ilford)
McVittie Anderson & Co., Ltd.
Sherman Chemicals Ltd.
Standard Synthetics Ltd.
Chas. Zimmermann & Co., Ltd.

TITANATE (BUTYL)
Titanium Intermediates Ltd.

TITANATE (ISOPROPYL)
Titanium Intermediates Ltd.

TITANATE (STEARYL)
Titanium Intermediates Ltd.

TITANATE (TRIETHANOLAMINE)
Titanium Intermediates Ltd.

TITANIUM DIOXIDE
D. F. Anstead Ltd.
British Titan Products Co., Ltd.
H. J. Evans & Co., Ltd.
The General Chemical Co., Ltd.
R. W. Greeff & Co., Ltd.
Geo. T. Gurr Ltd.
Laporte Industries Ltd. (Organics & Pigments Division–Stallingborough)
C. E. Ramsden & Co., Ltd.
Williams (Hounslow) Ltd.

TRIACETIN
Barter Trading Corporation Ltd.
Bush Boake Allen Ltd. Perfumery Division
Rex Campbell & Co., Ltd.
Croda Ltd.
Leek Chemicals Ltd.

TRICHLORETHYLENE
The General Chemical Co., Ltd.
Honeywill & Stein Ltd.
Imperial Chemical Industries Ltd.
Keegan Dyestuffs & Chemicals Ltd.
Kingsley & Keith (Chemicals) Ltd.
Sherman Chemicals Ltd.

TRIETHANOLAMINE

See also **Emulsifying agents**
Alwitt Ltd.
BASF United Kingdom Ltd.
Rex Campbell & Co., Ltd.
R. W. Greeff & Co., Ltd.
The General Chemical Co.,
  Ltd.
Hoechst Chemicals Ltd.
Honeywill & Stein Ltd.
Imperial Chemical Industries
  Ltd.
Kingsley & Keith (Chemicals)
  Ltd.
L. R. B. Pearce Ltd.
A. Revai & Co. (Chemicals),
  Ltd.
Shell Chemical U.K. Ltd.
Union Carbide Ltd. (Chemicals
  Division)

TRIPOLI POWDER

H. J. Evans & Co., Ltd.
Colin Stewart Ltd.

TRISODIUM PHOSPHATE *See* **Sodium phosphate, tribasic**

TURPENTINE

Berk Ltd.
British Celanese Ltd.
H. E. Daniel Ltd.
Fuerst Day Lawson Ltd.
A. V. Pound & Co., Ltd.
Smith & Forrest (Oils) Ltd.
Standard Synthetics Ltd.
White Sea & Baltic Co.,
  P. & I. Danischewsky Ltd.
Wynmouth Lehr & Fatoils Ltd.

TYLOSE

See **Cellulose methyl**

UMBELLIFERONE

See **Beta methyl umbelliferone**

UMBERS

See **Oxides, iron**

VALERIAN OIL

Bush Boake Allen Ltd.,
  Perfumery Division
Joseph Flach & Sons, Ltd.
H. Frischmann
John Kellys (London) Ltd.
R. Sarant & Co., Ltd.

VANILLIN

Bush Boake Allen Ltd.,

Perfumery Division
F. D. Copeland & Sons, Ltd.
Courtin & Warner Ltd.
H. E. Daniel Ltd.
Florasynth Ltd.
Food Industries Ltd.
Gale & Mount Ltd.
Givaudan & Co., Ltd.
The General Chemical Co.,
  Ltd.
R. W. Greeff & Co., Ltd.
Haarman & Reimer Ltd.
T. Harrison & Co., Ltd.
International Flavours &
  Fragrances I.F.F. (Gt.
  Britain) Ltd.
Monsanto Chemicals Ltd.
A. W. Munns & Co., Ltd.
Sherman Chemicals Ltd.
Söflor Ltd.
Standard Synthetics Ltd.
Chas. Zimmermann & Co.,
  Ltd.

VETIVERT OIL

V. Berg & Sons, Ltd.
Bertrand Freres Ltd.
Blyth, Greene & Jourdain &
  Co., Ltd.
Bush Boake Allen Ltd.,
  Perfumery Division
Charabot & Cie Ltd.
Antoine Chiris Ltd.
F. D. Copeland & Sons, Ltd.
H. E. Daniel Ltd.
Fuerst Day Lawson Ltd.
Gale & Mount Ltd.
A. J. Gomiero Ltd. (V. Mane
  Fils S.A.)
F. Gutkind & Co. Ltd.
Hollander Hyams Ltd.
Lautier Fils Ltd.
A. W. Munns & Co., Ltd.
Norda-Schimmel International
  Ltd.
Roure Bertrand Fils et Justin
  Dupont
P. Samuelson & Co., Ltd.
Standard Synthetics Ltd.
R. C. Treatt & Co., Ltd.
Alfred Paul White & Son
Wilson & Mansfield Ltd.

WAX (BEESWAX)

Bertrand Freres Ltd.
Victor Blagden & Co., Ltd.
British Wax Refining Co., Ltd.
Cyclo Chemicals Ltd.

Fuerst Day Lawson Ltd.
Geo. T. Gurr Ltd.
Holroyd's Oil & Ceresine Co.,
  Ltd.
Laing-National Ltd.
Poth, Hille & Co., Ltd.
Thew, Arnott & Co., Ltd.
Thews Ltd.
Wilkins, Campbell & Co., Ltd.
Harry B. Wood Ltd.
Wynmouth Lehr & Fatoils Ltd.

WAX (CARNAUBA)

Blyth, Greene Jourdain & Co.,
  Ltd.
British Wax Refining Co., Ltd.
Holroyd's Oil & Ceresine Co.
  Ltd.
Laing-National Ltd.
Poth, Hille & Co., Ltd.
Thew, Arnott & Co., Ltd.
Wilkins, Campbell & Co., Ltd.
Harry B. Wood Ltd.
Wynmouth Lehr & Fatoils Ltd.

WAX (CERESIN)

Astor, Boisselier & Lawrence
  Ltd.
British Wax Refining Co., Ltd.
Geo. T. Gurr Ltd.
Holroyd's Oil & Ceresine Co.
  Ltd.
Poth, Hille & Co., Ltd.
Thew, Arnott & Co., Ltd.
Wilkins, Campbell & Co., Ltd.
Harry B. Wood Ltd.
Wynmouth Lehr & Fatoils Ltd.

WAX, MICROCRYSTALLINE

Astor, Boisslier & Lawrence
  Ltd.
British Wax Refining Co., Ltd.
F. Chiesman & Co., Ltd.
Geo. T. Gurr Ltd.
Holroyd's Oil & Ceresine Co.
  Ltd.
Meade-King, Robinson & Co.,
  Ltd.
Poth, Hille & Co., Ltd.
Shell Chemical U.K. Ltd.
Thew, Arnott & Co., Ltd.
Wilkins, Campbell & Co., Ltd.
Harry B. Wood Ltd.
Wynmouth Lehr & Fatoils Ltd.

WAX (MONTAN)

British Wax Refining Co., Ltd.

Holroyd's Oil & Ceresine Co.
Ltd.
Poth, Hille & Co., Ltd.
Thew, Arnott & Co., Ltd.
Wilkins, Campbell & Co., Ltd.
Harry B. Wood Ltd.
Wynmouth Lehr & Fatoils Ltd.

WAX (PARAFFIN)
Astor, Boisselier & Lawrence
Ltd.
British Wax Refining Co., Ltd.
Guest Industrials Ltd.
Geo. T. Gurr Ltd.
Holroyd's Oil & Ceresine Co.
Ltd.
Laing-National Ltd.
Meade-King, Robinson & Co.,
Ltd.
L. R. B. Pearce Ltd.
Poth, Hille & Co., Ltd.
Shell Chemical U.K. Ltd.
Tar Residuals Ltd.
Thew, Arnott & Co., Ltd.
Thews Ltd.
Wilkins, Campbell & Co., Ltd.
Harry B. Wood Ltd.
Wynmouth Lehr & Fatoils Ltd.

WAXES (GENERAL)
See also **Wax, ozokerite**
Astor, Boisselier & Lawrence
Ltd.
British Wax Refining Co., Ltd.
Cornelius Produce Co., Ltd.
Fine Dyestuffs & Chemicals
Ltd.
Holroyd's Oil & Ceresine Co.
Ltd.
Meade-King, Robinson & Co.,
Ltd.
Poth, Hille & Co., Ltd.
Shell Chemical Co., Ltd.
Thew, Arnott & Co., Ltd.
Wilkins, Campbell & Co., Ltd.
Harry B. Wood Ltd.
Wynmouth Lehr & Fatoils Ltd.

WAXES, SYNTHETIC
Abril Industrial Waxes Ltd.
Astor, Boisselier & Lawrence
Ltd.
Bush Beach & Segner Bayley
Ltd.
Rex Campbell & Co., Ltd.
Cyclo Chemicals Ltd.
Dragoco (Gt. Britain) Ltd.
Dutton & Reinisch Ltd.

Fine Dyestuffs & Chemicals
Ltd.
Glovers (Chemicals) Ltd.
Hickson & Welch Ltd.
Hoechst Chemicals Ltd.
Holroyd's Oil & Ceresine Co.,
Ltd.
Kingsley & Keith (Chemicals)
Ltd.
Marchon Products Ltd.
Meade-King Robinson & Co.
Ltd.
Renham & Romley Ltd.
Ronsheim & Moore Ltd.
Sipon Products Ltd.
J. C. Thompson & Co. (Duron),
Ltd.
Union Carbide Ltd. (Chemicals
Division)
Wilkins, Campbell & Co., Ltd.
Victor Wolf Ltd.
Wynmouth Lehr & Fatoils Ltd.

WHEAT GERM OIL
Associated Preparations

WITCH HAZEL EXTRACT
Berk Ltd.
Bertrand Freres Ltd.
Bush Boake Allen Ltd.,
Perfumery Division
Dragoco (Gt. Britain) Ltd.
Joseph Flach & Sons, Ltd.
William Ransom & Son, Ltd.
Shearman & Co., Ltd.
Wilson & Mansfield.

WOOD WOOL
(*also* **Wood wool pads**)
Abbot's Packaging Ltd.
J. & W. Baldwin (Manchester)
Ltd.
W. B. C. (Packings) Ltd.
James Webster & Bro. Ltd.
Harry B. Wood Ltd.

WOOL FAT
Croda Ltd.
E. J. R. Lovelock
Meade-King Robinson & Co.
Ltd.
Pharmaceutical Co.
Westbrook Lanolin Co.
(Woolcombers) Ltd.
Harry B. Wood Ltd.

WOOL FAT DISTILLATES
Croda Ltd.
E. J. R. Lovelock

Westbrook Lanolin Co.
(Woolcombers), Ltd.
Victor Wolf Ltd.

WOOL GREASE
See also **Lanolin**
Croda Ltd.
M. Hamburger & Sons, Ltd.
E. J. R. Lovelock
Meade-King, Robinson & Co.,
Ltd.
Westbrook Lanolin Co.
(Woolcombers), Ltd.
Victor Wolf Ltd.
Wynmouth Lehr & Fatoils Ltd.

WOOL WAX
Croda Ltd.
Cyclo Chemicals Ltd.
Keegan Dyestuffs & Chemicals
Ltd.
Westbrook Lanolin Co.
(Woolcombers), Ltd.

XANTHOPHYLL
William Ransom & Son, Ltd.

YELLOW, VEGETABLE
See **Xanthophyll**

YLANG-YLANG OIL
Bertrand Freres Ltd.
Blyth, Greene & Jourdain &
Co., Ltd.
Bush Boake Allen Ltd.,
Perfumery Division
Charabot & Cie Ltd.
Antoine Chiris Ltd.
F. D. Copeland & Sons Ltd.
H. E. Daniel Ltd.
Dragoco (Gt. Britain) Ltd.
Felton Co. (Gt. Britain) Ltd.
Fuerst Day Lawson Ltd.
Gale & Mount Ltd.
A. J. Gomiero Ltd (V. Mane
Fils S.A.)
F. Gutkind & Co., Ltd.
W. H. Hobbs & Co., Ltd.
Lautier Fils Ltd.
Mallagh & Co.
A. W. Munns & Co., Ltd.
Natural & Synthetic Perfumery
Essence Co.
Norda-Schimmel International
Ltd.
P. T. Petley & Co., Ltd.
Roure Bertrand Fils et Justin
Dupont.
P. Samuelson & Co., Ltd.

R. Sarant & Co., Ltd.
Standard Synthetics Ltd.
H. E. Stringer Ltd.
R. C. Treatt & Co., Ltd.
Alfred Paul White & Son.
Wilson & Mansfield Ltd.
Chas. Zimmermann & Co.,
Ltd.

ZDRAVETS OIL
Bertrand Freres Ltd.
Charabot & Cie Ltd.
Wilson & Mansfield Ltd.

ZINC OXIDE
Dunn Bros. (Manchester) Ltd.
Durham Raw Materials Ltd.

H. J. Evans & Co., Ltd.
The General Chemical Co.,
Ltd.
R. W. Greeff & Co., Ltd.
Harrison, Clark Ltd.
Howards of Ilford Ltd.
Imperial Smelting Corporation
(N.S.C.) Ltd.
Millwards Merchandise Ltd.
Morris Ashby Ltd.
Thomas Morson & Son Ltd.
C. E. Ramsden & Co., Ltd.

ZINC PEROXIDE
The General Chemical Co.,
Ltd.

Laporte Industries Ltd.
(General Chemicals
Division–Luton)

ZINC STEARATE
Berk Ltd.
Bush Boake Allen Ltd.,
Perfumery Division
Dunn Bros., Manchester Ltd.
Durham Raw Materials Ltd.
Norman Evans & Rais Ltd.
The General Chemical Co.,
Ltd.
Hardman & Holden Ltd.
Thomas Morson & Son Ltd.
Wilfred Smith (Fine
Chemicals) Ltd.

The Boots Company Ltd., Consumer Products Development, Nottingham NG2 3AA (Boots the chemists), advise that the following items are likely to be available from their retail shops:

Acetone (commercial)
Almond oil BP
Arachis oil
Borax BP
Castor oil BP
Caustic soda
Citric acid
Coconut oil BPC
Corn oil
Epsom salts BP
Essence of peppermint BPC
Gelatin
Glycerin BP

Hydrogen peroxide solution
BP
Lanolin BP
Lavender oil
Lemon juice, unsweetened
Liquid paraffin BP
Magnesium carbonate, light BP
Milk, instant dried skimmed
Olive oil BP
Petroleum jelly
white BP
yellow BP
Purified water

Saccharin tablets BP
Sodium bicarbonate BP
Sodium sesquicarbonate BP
Starch
Surgical spirit BPC
Vinegar and cider vinegar
Vitamin C powder
Witch hazel, distilled BPC
Yeast

A

A.B.M. INDUSTRIAL PRODUCTS LTD.
Unity Mills, Poleacre Lane, Woodley,
Stockport, Cheshire and Bristol Road,
Gloucester.
ABRIL INDUSTRIAL WAXES LTD.
185 Aldersgate Street, London, E.C.1.
ADELPHI MANUFACTURING CO., LTD.
20–21 Duncan Terrace, London, N.1.
AEI – BIRLEC LTD.
Westgate, Aldridge, Staffordshire.
ALBION LABORATORIES LTD.
14–18 Talacre Rd., London, N.W.5.
ALBRIGHT & WILSON (MFG.) LTD.
1 Knightsbridge Green, London, S.W.1.
ALCOCK (PEROXIDE) LTD.
Leicester Road, Luton, Beds.
ALCOHOLS LTD.
48 Garman Road, London, N.17.
THE ALKA COMPANY
Maxwell Way, Gatwick Road, Crawley, Sussex.
**FREDERICK ALLEN & SONS
(CHEMICALS), LTD.**
Phoenix Chemical Works, Upper North St.,
London, E.14.
ALLEN DAVIES & CO., LTD.
Knapps Lane, St. George, Bristol 5.
ALLEN TRANSMATIC LTD.
28 Lyon Road, Hersham, Surrey.
**ALLIED COLLOIDS MANUFACTURING
CO., LTD.**
Cleckheaton Road, Low Moor, Bradford,
Yorks.
ALLUMINIUM CORPORATION LTD.
Bridgewater House, Cleveland Row, London,
S.W.1.
ALWITT LTD.
Zelide House, 2–4 Mount Ephraim, Tunbridge
Wells, Kent.
ANDREW & SUTER LTD.
Belmont Works, Belmont Hill, St. Albans,
Herts.
**ANGLO-SCOTTISH CHEMICAL CO.,
LTD.**
50 Wellington Street, Glasgow, C.2.
D. F. ANSTEAD LTD.
Victoria House, Radford Way, Billericay,
Essex.
THE A.P.V. CO., LTD.
Manor Royal, Crawley, Sussex.
ARENCO-ALITE LTD.
Pixmore Avenue, Letchworth, Herts.
ARMOUR HESS CHEMICALS LTD.
Westgate, Leeds 1, Yorks.
ARMSTRONG CORK CO., LTD.
Woodgrange House, Woodgrange Avenue,
Kenton, Middx.

AROMATICA LTD.
Sealand Road, Chester.
MORRIS ASHBY LTD.
10 Philpot Lane, London, E.C.3.
ASSOCIATED ADHESIVES LTD.
Knights Road, Silvertown, London, E.16.
**ASSOCIATED CHEMICAL COMPANIES
(Mfg.) LTD.**
Beckwith Knowle, Otley Road, Harrogate,
Yorks.
ASSOCIATED PREPARATIONS
P.O. Box 53, Cheam, Surrey.
**ASTOR, BOISSELIER & LAWRENCE
LTD.**
1 Lancaster Place, Strand, London, W.C.2.
ATKINS & CO.
19 Hardres Street, Ramsgate, Kent.
AUSTIN & CO. (CONTAINERS), LTD.
Cole Kings, Hagden Lane, Watford, Herts.
W. R. F. AVERY & CO.
245 New Kings Road, London, S.W.6.

B

BABCOCK & WILCOX LTD.
209 Euston Road, London, N.W.1.
BACTEROL LTD.
Old Powder Mills Depot, Leigh, Nr.
Tonbridge, Kent.
**BAIRD & TATLOCK GROUP OF
COMPANIES**
18 Great Marlborough Street, London, W.1.
and M. & B. Works, Blackhorse Lane, London,
E.17.
BAKELITE XYLONITE LTD.
Cascelloid Division, P.O. Box 103, Abbey
Lane, Leicester.
PERCY P. BAKER LTD.
28–36 Orsman Road, London, N.1.
BAKER PERKINS HOLDINGS LTD.
Westwood Works, Peterborough.
RICHARD BAKER & CO., LTD.
12 Broadway, London, S.W.1.
J. & W. BALDWIN (MANCHESTER) LTD.
Mellors Road, Trafford Park, Manchester, 17.
HENRY BALFOUR & CO. LTD.
Artillery House, Artillery Row, London,
S.W.1.
BANISTER STREET WORKS LTD.
175 Lower Clapton Road, London, E.5.
J. BARCHAM GREEN LTD.
Hayle Mill, Maidstone, Kent.
HENRY BARLOW & SONS (OILS), LTD.
Belmont Oil Works, Lancashire Hill, Stockport,
Cheshire.
JACK L. BARNETT LTD.
12 Meadow Lane, Leeds, Yorks.

R. W. BARRACLOUGH LTD.
1 Hartwood Road, Southport, Lancs.
BARTER TRADING CORPORATION LTD.
69 Grosvenor Street, London, W.1.
BARTHES-ROBERTS LTD.
59 Lant Street, London, S.E.1.
BARTOLINE (HULL) LTD.
Triumph Works, Air St., Hull, Yorks.
BASF UNITED KINGDOM LTD.
York House, 199 Westminster Bridge Road, London, S.E.1.
BEATSON, CLARK & CO., LTD.
Rotherham, Yorks.
BELLINGHAM & STANLEY LTD.
61 Markfield Road, London, N.15.
V. BERG & SONS, LTD.
Colonial House, Mark Lane, London, E.C.3.
BERK LTD.
Berk House, P.O. Box 1BL., 8 Baker Street, London, W.1.
BERK SPENCER ACIDS LTD.
Abbey Mills Chemical Works, Stratford, London, E.15.
BERTRAND FRERES LTD.
P.O. Box 1D7, Hesketh House, Portman Square, London, W.1.
BERSEL MFG. CO., LTD.
Lawrence Works, West Green Road, Tottenham, N.15.
BESPAK INDUSTRIES LTD.
Acos Works, Eleanor Cross Road, Waltham Cross, Herts.
BETTIX LTD.
Dunbar Road, New Malden, Surrey.
BETTS & CO., LTD.
Holloway Mills, Elthorne Road, London, N.19.
BIBBY & BARON CARTONS LTD.
Hardys Gate, Dumers Lane, Bury, Lancs.
J. BIBBY & SONS, LTD.
King Edward St., Liverpool 3.
BILIPAK LTD.
10 Radford Cresent, Billericay, Essex.
BIO-COSMETIC RESEARCH LABORATORIES
128 High Street, Edgware, Middx.
BIRMINGHAM CHEMICAL CO., LTD.
St. John's St., Lichfield, Staffs.
VICTOR BLAGDEN & CO., LTD.
Plantation House, Mincing Lane, London, E.C.3.
BLAIRS LTD.
Glasgow Engineering Works, 143 Woodville St., Glasgow, S.W.1.
BLUNDELL & CROMPTON LTD.
West India Dock Road, London, E.14.

BLYTH, GREENE, JOURDAIN & CO., LTD.
Plantation House, Fenchurch St., London, E.C.3.
W. BLYTHE & CO., LTD.
Holland Bank Chemical Works, Church, Lancs.
BOARD PRODUCTS LTD.
Montrose Street, Fenton, Stoke-on-Trent.
FREDK. BOEHM LTD.
19 Bentinck St., W.1.
JOHN BOND (LONDON) LTD.
74 Southgate Road, London, N.1.
J. BOOTH & SON, LTD.
Canal Wharf, Canal Road, Congleton, Cheshire.
JOHN BOOTH & SONS (BOLTON), LTD.
Hulton Steelworks, Bolton.
BORAX & CHEMICALS LTD.
35 Piccadilly, London, W.1.
BORAX CONSOLIDATED LTD.
Borax House, Carlisle Place, London, S.W.1.
BOWMANS CHEMICALS LTD.
P.O. Box No. 10, Moss Bank, Widnes, Lancs.
BOWRING, JONES & TIDY LTD.
52, Leadenhall St., London, E.C.3.
FREDK. BRABY & CO., LTD.
Braby House, Smithfield St., London, E.C.1.
BRAMIGK & CO., LTD.
31–35 Wilson Street, London, E.C.2.
S. BRAMWELL & CO., LTD.
246–252 Produce Exchange, Manchester 4.
BRATBY & HINCHLIFFE LTD.
Gorton Lane, Manchester 18.
BRENT MANUFACTURING CO.
Commerce Road, Brentford, Middx.
BRENTFORD SOAP CO., LTD.
Brent Works, Brentford, Middx.
WM. BRIERLEY COLLIER & HARTLEY LTD.
Boro Works, Bridgefield St., Rochdale, Lancs.
S. BRIGGS & CO., LTD.
P.O. Box 6, New Street, Burton-on-Trent.
BRITISH ANHYDROUS AMMONIA CO., LTD.
Magdala Works, 518 Woolwich Road, London, S.E.7.
BRITISH CELANESE LTD.
Chemicals & Plastics Group, 345 Foleshill Road, Coventry.
BRITISH CELILYND LTD.
97 Lea Bridge Road, London, E.10.
BRITISH DRUG HOUSES LTD., THE,
BDH Laboratory Chemicals Division, Poole, Dorset.
BRITISH OIL & CAKE MILLS LTD.
St. Bridget's House, Bridewell Place, London, E.C.4.

BRITISH OXYGEN CO., LTD.
Hammersmith House, London, W.6.
BRITISH RAYOPHANE LTD.
11 New Fetter Lane, London, E.C.4.
BRITISH REMA MFG. CO., LTD.
1 Industry Road, Sheffield 9, Yorks.
BRITISH RESIN PRODUCTS LTD.
Devonshire House, Piccadilly, London, W.1.
BRITISH SIDAC LTD.
Hesketh House, Portman Square, London, W.1.
BRITISH TITAN PRODUCTS CO., LTD.
10 Stratton St., London, W.1.
THE BRITISH WAX REFINING CO. LTD.
31 St. John's Road, Redhill, Surrey.
BROTHERTON & CO., LTD.
Nechells Chemical Works, Birmingham 7.
BROWN & FORTH LTD.
Clifton House, 83–117 Euston Road, London, N.W.1.
BROWN & SON (ALEMBIC WORKS), LTD.
9 Wedmore Street, London, N.19.
BRUCE & HYSLOP LTD.
Well Lane, off Park Street, Bootle, 20, Lancs.
BRUCE, STARKE & CO., LTD.
Ashley House, 96 Hatton Garden, London, E.C.1.
BUELL LTD.
8/10 Minerva Road, North Acton, London, N.W.10.
BUHLER BROS.
The Wood House, Cockfosters, Barnet, Herts.
BURMAH OIL TRADING LTD.
Lobitos Division, 76 Jermyn Street, London, S.W.1.
R. H. BURMAN LTD.
897 Tyburn Road, Erdington, Birmingham 24.
JAMES BURROUGH LTD.
Vauxhall Street, Lambeth, London, S.E.11.
BUSH BEACH & SEGNER BAYLEY LTD.
Marlow House, Lloyds Avenue, London, E.C.3.
BUSH BOAKE ALLEN LTD.
(Overseas Sales) Flavour Division, Ash Grove, Hackney, London, E.8.
BUSH BOAKE ALLEN LTD.
Perfumery Division, Blackhorse Lane, Walthamstow, London, E.17.
BUSH BOAKE ALLEN LTD.
(U.K. Sales) Flavour Division, Wharf Road, London, N.1.
W. P. BUTTERFIELD LTD.
P.O. Box 38, Shipley, Yorks.
BUTTERFIELD LABORATORIES LTD.
Carpenters Road, Stratford, London, E.15.

C

CAMILLI ALBERT & LALOUE
Grasse (A.M.), France.
REX CAMPBELL & CO., LTD.
7 Idol Lane, London, E.C.3.
CANNON INDUSTRIES LTD.
Deepfields, Nr. Bilston, Staffs.
CARESSA LTD.
527/539 Harrow Road, London, W.10.
CARLSON-FORD SALES LTD.
Newman Street, Ashton under Lyne, Lancs.
CARR & CO. (PAPER), LTD.
Carco Mills, Shirley, Solihull, Warwicks.
CARTY & SON, LTD.
Harders Road, Peckham, London, S.E.15.
CASEIN (INDUSTRIES) LTD.
20 Linford Street, London, S.W.8.
CASTROL LTD.
Castrol House, Marylebone Road, London, N.W.1.
CHALK PRODUCTS LTD.
138 Sloane Street, London, S.W.1.
CHARABOT & CIE LTD.
90–92 Great Portland Street, London, W.1.
CHEMICAL & INSULATING CO. LTD.
Darlington, Co. Durham.
CHESHIRE GELATINES
Sutton Weater, Near Warrington.
MAURICE CHEVALIER
U.K. Agent-'UNIVER', 24 High Holborn, London, W.C.1.
F. CHIESMAN & CO., LTD.
1 Fenchurch Buildings, Fenchurch St., London, E.C.3.
ANTOINE CHIRIS LTD.
39 East Street, Epsom, Surrey.
CIBA AEROCHEMICALS LTD.
'Killgerm' Disenfectant Division, P.O. Box 1, Mirfield, Yorks.
CIBA CLAYTON LTD.
571 Ashton New Rd., Clayton, Manchester 11.
CHARLES CLAY & SONS LTD.
53 Cheapside, Luton, Beds.
GEO. S. CLAYTON LTD.
St. Anne's Works, St. Anne St., London, E.4.
WILLIAM W. CLELAND LTD.
Staple House, Chancery Lane, London, W.C.2.
COALITE & CHEMICAL PRODUCTS LTD.
P.O. Box 21, Chesterfield, Derbyshire.
COCHRAN & CO. (ANNAN), LTD.
23 Strutton Ground, S.W.1.
COCKER CHEMICAL CO. LTD.
Nook Lane, Oswaldtwistle, Nr. Accrington, Lancs.

204

GEORGE COHEN, SONS & CO., LTD.
Stanningly, Nr. Leeds, Yorks.
COLGATE PALMOLIVE LTD.
317 Ordsall Lane, Manchester 5.
COLLINGHAM & OWEN LTD.
Windsor St., Beeston, Nottinghamshire.
THOMAS COLLINS & CO. LTD.
21–37 Barclay Place, Edinburgh, 10.
COLNE VALE DYE & CHEMICAL CO.,
LTD.
Milnsbridge, Huddesfield, Yorks.
COLODENSE LTD.
West St., Bristol 3.
COLUMBIAN INTERNATIONAL (GT.
BRITAIN) LTD.
116 Cannon Street, London, E.C.4.
FRANK A. CONDUIT & CO.,
6 Snow Hill, London, E.C.1.
ALFRED CONNER & CO., LTD.
Fife Street, Nuneaton, Warwickshire.
CONTINENTAL OIL CO., LTD.
Conoco Petrochemicals Division, Berkeley
Square House, Berkeley Square, London, W.1.
CO-OPERATIVE WHOLESALE
SOCIETY LTD.
Irlam, Manchester.
F. D. COPELAND & SONS LTD.
115 Gray's Inn Road, London, W.C.1.
BRYAN CORCORAN LTD.
Westminster Bank Chambers, 130 Whitechapel
High St., London, E.1.
CORFIELD & BUCKLE LTD.
Trafalgar Works, Station Road, Merton Abbey,
London, S.W.19.
CORN PRODUCTS (SALES) LTD.
Claygate House, Esher, Surrey.
CORNELIUS PRODUCE CO., LTD.
Ibex House, Minories, London, E.C.3.
CORNWELL PRODUCTS LTD.
56–60 Hallam St., London, W.1.
COURTAULDS LTD.
22 Hanover Square, London, W.1.
COURTIN & WARNER LTD.
Ballards Old Brewery, Bell Lane, Lewes,
Sussex.
E. COWLES LTD.
Whiffler Road, Drayton Road Industrial Estate,
Norwich.
CRODA LTD.
Cowick Hall, Snaith, Goole, Yorks.
JOSEPH CROSFIELD & SONS, LTD.
Bank Quay Works, Warrington, Lancs.
CULLINGFORD OF CHELSEA.
Lunt Avenue, Bootle 10, Lancs.
J. W. CUMMING & SON, LTD.
Cow Lane Works, Oldfield Road, Salford 5,

Lancs., and 66/70 Borough High Street,
London, S.E.1.
CUNDELL, EVE & CO., LTD.
Old Ford Works, Smeed Road, London, E.3.
CYCLO CHEMICALS LTD.
Nathan Way, Woolwich Industrial Estate,
London, S.E.18.

D

JOHN DALE LTD.
Brunswick Park Road, New Southgate,
London, N.11.
H. E. DANIEL LTD.
Longfield Road, North Farm Industrial Estate,
Tunbridge Wells, Kent.
DANKS OF NETHERTON LTD.
P.O Box 22, Netherton, Dudley, Worcs.
DAVEY, PAXMAN & CO., LTD.
P.O. Box No. 8, Colchester, Essex.
DAVIDSON & CO., LTD.
Sirocco Engineering Works, Belfast, 5.
JOHN DEIGHTON & CO., LTD.
11 Grape Lane, Petergate, York.
W. M. DELF (LIVERPOOL) LTD.
Delco Works, Rice Lane, Liverpool 9.
DELITTLE FENWICK & CO., LTD.
Railway St., York.
W. M. R. DELL & SON, LTD.
48 Weston St., London, S.E.1.
DENNISON MANUFACTURING CO.,
LTD.
Colonial Way, Watford, Herts.
DEWRANCE-TRIANGLE LTD.
33–39 Saville Row, London, W.1.
JOHN DICKINSON & CO., LTD. (DRG
COMPANY)
Apsley Mills, Hemel Hempstead, Herts.
DISTILLERS CO., LTD.
Devonshire House, Piccadilly, London, W.1.
DISTILLERS CHEMICALS & PLASTICS
LTD.
Industrial Solvents Division, Devonshire
House, Mayfair Place, Piccadilly, London, W.1.
DIVERSEY LTD.
Cockfosters, Barnet, Herts.
DOBEY LTD.
260 High Road, Tottenham, N.15.
JOHN DORE & CO., LTD.
Fowler Road, Hainault, Ilford, Essex.
DRAGOCO (GT. BRITAIN) LTD.
Tallon Road, Brentwood, Essex.
DRIVER SOUTHALL LTD.
Villa St. Works, Hockley, Birmingham 19.
DRUMS LTD.
Grosvenor Gardens House, London, S.W.1.

DUBUIS & ROWSELL LTD.
Duroma Works, Elmwood Road, Croydon, CR9
2TX, Surrey.
T. M. DUCHE & SONS (U.K.), LTD.
Adelaide House, London Bridge, London,
E.C.4.
DUNLOP CO., LTD.
10 King Street, St. James's, London, S.W.1.
DUNN BROS. MANCHESTER LTD.
Bowlee Mill, 382 Heywood Old Road, Bowlee,
Middleton. Manchester.
DU PONT CO. (U.K.) LTD.
18 Breams Buildings, Fetter Lane, London,
E.C.4.
DURHAM RAW MATERIALS LTD.
1–4 Great Tower St., London, E.C.3.
LEONARD DUTTON & SONS
2 Salmon Lane, London, E.14.
DUTTON & REINISCH LTD.
132 Cromwell Road, London, S.W.7.

E

EAST LANCASHIRE CHEMICAL CO., LTD.
Fairfield Road, Droylsden, Manchester.
EDIPRO LTD.
Petrofina House, York Road, London, S.E.1.
A. ELDER REED & CO., LTD.
Riverside House, Carnwath Rd., London, S.W.6.
ELGA PRODUCTS LTD.
Lane End, Bucks.
H. J. ELLIOTT LTD.
E-Mil Works, Treforest Industrial Estate,
Nr. Pontypridd, Glam.
B. ELLIS & CO., LTD.
9–13 Pleasant Hill St., Liverpool 8.
ELLIS JONES & CO. (STOCKPORT), LTD.
Tiviot Colour Works, Stockport, Cheshire.
EMHART (U.K.) LTD.
Crompton Road, Wheatley, Doncaster, Yorks.
EMMERICH (LONDON) LTD.
Derbyshire House, St. Chad's Street,
King's Cross, London, W.C.1.
ENGLISH CLAYS LOVERING POCHIN & CO., LTD.
John Keay House, St. Austell, Cornwall.
H. ERBEN LTD.
185A Brompton Road, London, S.W.3.
EVANS CHEMICALS LTD.
Boreham Wood, Herts.
H. J. EVANS & CO., LTD.
222A Allerton Road, Liverpool 18.
NORMAN EVANS & RAIS LTD.
Woodley, Stockport, Cheshire.

F

M. J. FECHER LTD.
Littlefield Works, 175 Bath Road, Slough, Bucks.
WALTER H. FELTHAM & SON, LTD.
49/61 Pancras Road, London, N.W.1.
FELTON COMPANY (GREAT BRITAIN) LTD.
White Lodge, Hampton Court Road,
East Molesey, Surrey
FIBRENYLE LTD.
Skylon House, Gosford Road, Beccles, Suffolk.
WM. FIDDES & SON, LTD.
Torry Sawmills, Aberdeen.
FIELD & CO. (AROMATICS), LTD.
Stonefield Close, Ruislip, Middx.
FINE DYESTUFFS & CHEMICALS LTD.
Calder Street, Manchester 2.
FIRMENICH LTD.
414 London Road, Isleworth, Middx.
FISCHER & PORTER LTD.
Salterbeck Trading Estate, Workington,
Cumberland.
JOSEPH FLACH & SONS, LTD.
140 Falkland Road, Harringay, London, N.8.
FLORASYNTH LTD.
327–347 Oldfield Lane, Greenford, Middx.
FORDS (FINSBURY) LTD.
Chantry Avenue, Kempston, Bedford.
R. FOSTER & CO. (DISPLAY) LTD.
Arfrosta House, Uxbridge Road, London, W.7.
SAMUEL FOX & CO., LTD.
Stocksbridge Works, Sheffield.
FRENCH FLINT & ORMCO LTD.
Ibex House, Minories, London, E.C.3.
H. FRISCHMANN
16 North End Road, London, N.W.1.
FUERST DAY LAWSON LTD.
1 Leadenhall Street, London, E.C.3.
FULLERS' EARTH UNION LTD.
Patterson Court, Nutfield Road, Redhill, Surrey.

G

GALE & MOUNT LTD.
Commerce House, Commerce Road, Brentford,
Middx.
A. GALLENKAMP & CO., LTD.
Christopher Street, London, E.C.2.
HARRY H. GARDAM & CO., LTD.
100 Church St., Staines, Middx.
GARDNERS OF GLOUCESTER
Winglos House, Bristol Road, Gloucester.
GEIGY (U.K.) LIMITED
Simonsway, Manchester 22.
THE GENERAL CHEMICAL CO., LTD.
Judex Works, Sudbury, Wembley, Middx.

GENT & CO. LIMITED
Faraday Works, Leicester.
GERARD-POLYSULPHIN LTD.
Wilkinson Street, New Basford, Nottingham.
GERMSTROYD PRODUCTS LTD.
Anchor Works, 50 Raphael St., Bolton, Lancs.
J. A. GILBURT LTD.
Elsden Mews, Old Ford Road, Bethnal Green,
London, E.2.
T. GIUSTI & SON, LTD.
202–224 York Way, London, N.7.
GIVAUDAN & CO., LTD.
Godstone Road, Whyteleafe, Surrey. CR3 0YE
GLASTICS LTD.
9 Salisbury Road, Barnet, Herts.
GLOVERS (CHEMICALS) LTD.
Wortley Low Mills, Whitehall Road, Leeds 12,
Yorks.
GLYCERINE LTD.
Hesketh House, Portman Square, London, W.1.
GOLDEN VALLEY COLOURS LTD.
Wick, Bristol.
A. J. GOMIERO LTD. (V. MANE FILS S.A.)
Unit No. 12, 8 Andrews Road, London, E.8.
GOODYEAR TYRE & RUBBER CO., LTD.
Stewart Street, Wolverhampton, Staffs.
**EDWARD GORTON LTD. (CHESHIRE
GELATINES BRANCH)**
Sutton Weaver, Warrington, Lancs.
JOHN GOSHERON & CO., LTD.
58 Kensington Church St., London, W.8.
JOHN GOSNELL & CO., LTD.
Southover, Lewes, Sussex.
R. W. GREEFF & CO., LTD.
31–45 Gresham St., London, E.C.2.
N. GREENING & SONS, LTD.
Britannia Works, Bewsey Road, Warrington.
JAMES GREENSHIELDS & CO., LTD.
258 Bath St., Glasgow, C.2.
GRIFFIN & GEORGE LTD.
Ealing Road, Alperton, Wembley, Middx.
A. F. GROVER & CO., LTD.
Higham Road, Chesham, Bucks.
GUEST INDUSTRIALS LTD.
81 Gracechurch St., London, E.C.3.
GULF OIL (GREAT BRITAIN) LTD.
6 Grosvenor Place, London, S.W.1.
GEO. T. GURR LTD.
136–144 New King's Road, London, S.W.6.
F. GUTKIND & CO. LTD.
82 King William St., London, E.C.4.

H

HAARMAN & REIMER LTD.
Kingsway House, 18–24 Paradise Road,
Richmond, Surrey.
ROBERT HALDANE & CO., LTD.
Underwood Chemical Works, Murray St.,
Paisley, Scotland.
M. HAMBURGER & SONS, LTD.
Plantation House, Mincing Lane, London, E.C.3.
HANSON & EDWARDS LTD.
Vernon St., Warrington, Lancs.
HARCOSTAR LTD.
Windover Road, Huntingdon.
HARDMAN & HOLDEN LTD.
'Manox' House, Coleshill Street, Miles Platting,
Manchester 10.
F. & R. M. HARRIS (B'HAM) LTD.
Chemix Buildings, Dudley Road, Halesowen,
Birmingham.
HARRIS HART & CO., LTD.
Gregge Street Works, Heywood, Lancs.
**GEO. H. HARRISON & SONS (LEEDS),
LTD.**
Statue Printing Works, Lovell Road, Leeds 7.
T. HARRISON & CO., LTD.
Burnley House, Willesden, London, N.W.10.
W. HARRISON & CO. LTD.
12 Broadway, London, S.W.1.
HARRISON CLARK LTD.
391 Dickenson Road, Longsight, Manchester 13.
HARTLEY & SUGDEN LTD.
White Rose Boiler Works, Halifax, Yorks.
HARVEY FABRICATION LTD.
Woolwich Road, London, S.E.7.
W. HAWLEY & SON, LTD.
Colour Works, Duffield, Derby. DE6 4FG
HERCULES POWDER CO., LTD.
1 Gt. Cumberland Place, London, W.1.
A. G. HERSOM
123 Richmond Road, Kingston-Upon-Thames,
Surrey.
RENE HEYMANS LTD.
12–14 Middle St., London, E.C.1.
HICKSON & WELCH LTD.
Ings Lane, Castleford, Yorks.
M. AGUSTI HIDALGO (LONDON) LTD.
81 Ledbury Road, London, W.11
HIGHGATE & JOB LTD.
60 Murray Street, Paisley, Scotland, and
Regent Road, Liverpool 5.
HILGER & WATTS LTD.
98 St. Pancras Way, London, N.W.1.
HIRON & REMPLER LTD.
32–36 St. Anne St., London, E.14.
**A. HIRSCH (FILTERIT) LTD. NOW
BRITISH FILTERS LTD.**

W. HITCHINS (1932) LTD.
51–57 High Street South, East Ham,
London, E.6.
W. H. HOBBS & CO., LTD.
166 Tower Bridge Road, London, S.E.1.
HOECHST CHEMICALS LTD.
Hoechst House, Kew Bridge, Brentford, Middx.
HOLDEN & BROOKE LTD.
Sirius Works, Manchester 12.
HOLLANDER HYAMS LTD.
20–22 Bedford Row, London, W.C.1.
HOLLANDS DISTILLERY (ESSENTIAL OILS) LTD.
37 Wood Street, Mitcham Junction, Surrey.
CR4 4JT
HOLPAK LTD.
Bessemer Road, Welwyn Garden City, Herts.
HOLROYD'S OIL & CERESINE CO., LTD.
37 High Street, Stratford, London, E.15.
HONEYWILL & STEIN LTD.
Devonshire House, Mayfair Place, London, W.1.
G. HOPKINS & SONS, LTD.
United House, North Road, London, N.7.
HOPKINSONS LTD.
P.O. Box B.27, Huddersfield, Yorks.
HOWARDS OF ILFORD LTD.
Uphall Road, Ilford, Essex.
HULL CHEMICAL WORKS LTD.
Kirkby St., Hull, Yorks.
G. C. HURRELL & CO., LTD.
Knight Road, Strood, Rochester, Kent.
HUSSEY GWENDA PRODUCTS LTD.
Gwenda Works, Legge Lane, Birmingham, 1.

I

IMPAG (LONDON) LTD.
10 Lloyds Avenue, London, E.C.3.
IMPERIAL CHEMICAL INDUSTRIES LTD.
Imperial Chemical House, Millbank, London,
S.W.1.
J. K. INNES & CO., LTD.
Kingmoor Works, Kingmoor Road, Carlisle,
Cumberland.
INSULL & POINTON LTD.
St. Mary's Engineering Works, Tunstall,
Stoke-on-Trent, Staffs.
INTERNATIONAL COMBUSTION PRODUCTS LTD.
19 Woburn Place, London, W.C.1.
INTERNATIONAL FLAVOURS & FRAGRANCES I.F.F. (GT. BRITAIN) LTD.
Crown Road, off Southbury Road, Enfield,
Middx.

ISOPAD LTD.
Barnet By-Pass, Boreham Wood, Herts.
IVERS-LEE (G.B.) LTD.
Cordwallis Estate, Cookham Road, Maidenhead,
Berks.

J

J. G. JACKSON & CROCKATT LTD.
Nitshill Road, Thornlie bank, Glasgow.
JOHN P. JACKSON & CO., LTD.
47a Marlborough St., Liverpool 3.
JACOBSON VAN DEN BERG & CO. (U.K.) LTD.
Jacoberg House, Emerald Street, London,
W.C.1.
JAHN (MASKINER) LTD.
34 York Way, Kings Cross, London, N.1.
ROBERT JENKINS & CO., LTD.
Ivanhoe Works, Wortley Road, Rotherham,
Yorks.
JENNER & GILL LTD.
Landor Street, Birmingham 8.
JESSOP & CO.
10 Cullum Street, London, E.C.3.
JEYES GROUP LTD.
31 River Road, Barking, Essex.
F. G. JOHNS & Co., LTD.
Escalia Works, Argall Avenue, London, E.10.
JOHNS-MANVILLE (GT. BRITAIN) LTD.
20 Albert Embankment, London, S.E.1.
JOHNSEN & JORGENSEN LTD.
Herringham Road, Charlton, London, S.E.7.
A. JOHNSON & CO. (LONDON), LTD.
Molly Millars Lane, Wokingham, Berks.
JOHNSON MATTHEY CHEMICALS LTD.
74 Hatton Garden, London, E.C.1.
S. H. JOHNSON & CO., LTD.
Carpenters Road, Stratford, London, E.15.
SAMUEL JONES & CO., LTD.
Butterfly House, Dingwall Road, Croydon,
CR9 3DA.
C. H. G. JOURDAN LTD.
27 Maddox Street, London, W.1.

K

L. KAHN MANUFACTURING CO., LTD.
527–539 Harrow Road, London, W.10.
KEEGAN DYESTUFFS & CHEMICALS LTD.
164 Garnett St., Bradford, Yorks.
KEITH BLACKMAN LTD.
Mill Mead Road, London, N.17.
KEK LTD.
Palmerston St., Ancoats, Manchester 12.

208

ROBERT KELLIE & SON, LTD.
40 East Dock Street, Dundee, Scotland.
JOHN KELLYS (LONDON) LTD.
Ibex House, Minories, London, E.C.3.
KIMBERLY-CLARK LTD.
Larkfield, Nr. Maidstone, Kent.
KING (M.T.D.), LTD.
19 Grosvenor Place, London, S.W.1.
C. E. KING & SONS LTD.
41 London Street, Chertsey, Surrey.
KINGSLEY & KEITH (CHEMICALS) LTD.
73–76 Jermyn Street, London, S.W.1.
KOLMAR COSMETICS (ENGLAND) LTD.
Felbridge Laboratories, Imberhorne Lane, East Grinstead, Sussex.
KONINGEN LTD.
Park Garden Factory, Pembroke Gardens, Park Street, Camberley, Surrey.

L

LAING-NATIONAL LTD.
24 Mosley Street, Manchester 2.
LAM GROUP
37 Peter Street, Manchester 2.
LAMBOURNES (B'HAM) LTD.
Gt. Hampton Works, Birmingham 19.
LANCASHIRE TAR DISTILLERS LTD.
P.O. Box 453, Corporation St., Manchester 4.
LANCASTER & TONGE LTD.
The Lancaster Works, Pendleton, Manchester 6.
JULES LANG & SON
Farringdon Station Chambers, Cowcross St., London, E.C.1.
LANG-LONDON LTD.
Southall Lane, Hounslow, Middx.
LANGLEY SMITH & CO., LTD.
19–21 Christopher St., London, E.C.2.
H. M. LANGTON & CO., LTD.
8 Bloomsbury Square, London, W.C.1.
LANKRO CHEMICALS LTD.
Bentcliffe Works, Salters Lane, Eccles, Manchester.
LAPORTE INDUSTRIES LTD., GENERAL CHEMICALS DIVISION
Moorfield Road, Widnes, Lancs., and P.O. Box 8, Luton, Beds., and 10 Eastgate, Leeds 2, and P.O. Box 7, Warrington Lancs.
ORGANICS & PIGMENTS DIVISION
Stallingborough, Lincs., and Nutfield Road, Redhill, Surrey, and Uphall Road, Ilford, Essex.

LEOPOLD LASERSON LTD.
37 Rothschild Road, London, W.4.
LAUGHTON & SONS, LTD.
Warstock Road, Birmingham 14.
LAUTIER FILS LTD.
Power Road, Chiswick, London, W.4.
LAWTONS OF LIVERPOOL LTD.
60 Vauxhall Road, Liverpool 3.
LEEK CHEMICALS LTD.
Bridge End Works, Leek, Staffs.
WALTER LEHMANN
92 Caledonian Road, Kings Cross, London, N.W.1.
LENNIG CHEMICALS LTD.
26–28 Bedford Row, London, W.C.1.
A. LEVERMORE & CO., LTD.
Broadway House, Broadway, Wimbledon, London, S.W.19.
LIME-FREE WATER & GENERAL SERVICES LTD.
Grosvenor Gardens House, London, S.W.1.
LIVERPOOL BORAX CO., LTD. NOW L.T.D. BUILDING PRODUCTS
6 St. Paul's Square, Liverpool 3.
LOCKER INDUSTRIES LTD.
Church Street, Warrington, Lancs.
LOCKWOOD MAGRATH PTY., LTD.
P.O. Box 50, Botany, N.S.W. 2019, Australia.
S. C. LOMAX LTD.
Alfreds Way, Barking, Essex.
LONDON ALUMINIUM CO., LTD.
Bridgnorth Road, Wombourn, Wolverhampton.
LONDON TAR & CHEMICAL CO., LTD.
Corn Exchange Building, 52/57 Mark Lane, London, E.C.3.
E. J. R. LOVELOCK
Oaklands House, Oaklands Drive, Sale, Manchester.
LOWE & CARR LTD.
Liberty Works, Eastern Boulevard, Leicester.
L.T.D. BUILDING PRODUCTS (DETERGENTS SECTION) A division of Lancashire Tar Distillers Ltd.
6 St. Paul's Square, Liverpool 3.
LUNEVALE PRODUCTS LTD.
Low Mill, Halton, Lancaster.
PETER LUNT & CO., LTD.
Park Lane, Aintree, Liverpool 10.
W. LUSTY & SONS, LTD.
Bromley-by-Bow, London, E.3.

M

McKIE & BAXTER LTD.
Copland Works, Murray St., Paisley, Scotland.
GERALD McDONALD & CO., LTD.
9 Botolph Lane, London, E.C.3.
McVITTIE ANDERSON & CO., LTD.
20–22 Bedford Row, London, W.C.1.
MALLAGH & CO.
17 Carnarvon Road, South Woodford, London, E.18.
MANLOVE, ALLIOTT & CO., LTD.
P.O. Box 81, Bloomsgrove Works, Nottingham.
A. J. MANNING LTD.
Stonefield Close, South Ruislip, Middx.
MARCHANT BROS. LTD.
60 Verney Road, London, S.E.16.
MARCHON PRODUCTS LTD.
Whitehaven, Cumberland.
MARSHALL, SONS & CO., LTD.
Britannia Works, Gainsborough, Lincs.
MATTHEWS, SMITH & CO., LTD.
Digby Works, Homerton High St., London, E.9.
MATTHEWS & YATES LTD.
Cyclone Works, Swinton, Manchester.
MAY & BAKER LTD.
Dagenham, Essex.
MEADE-KING, ROBINSON & CO., LTD.
Tower Building, Liverpool 3.
P. MELLIS & SONS
8 Elder St., Bishopsgate, London, E.1.
METHYLATING CO., LTD.
Devonshire House, Mayfair Place, London, W.1.
MIDLAND SILICONES LTD.
Reading Bridge House, Reading, Berks.
MIDLAND TAR DISTILLERS LTD.
Springfield Chemical Works, Oldbury, Birmingham.
MIKROPUL LTD.
40 Towerfield Road, Shoeburyness, Essex.
J. & G. MILLER
37–39 Wood Street, Mitcham Junction, Surrey. CR4 4JT.
MIRACLE MILLS LTD.
90 Lots Road, Chelsea, London, S.W.10.
MIRVALE CHEMICAL CO., LTD.
Mirfield, Yorks.
C. MITCHELL & CO., LTD. Agents for BASF A.G.
1–3 Snow Hill, London, E.C.1.
T. M. MOCKRIDGE & CO.
52 Tanner Street, Hyde, Cheshire.
MONSANTO CHEMICALS LTD.
10–18 Victoria St., London, S.W.1.
MORGAN FAIREST LTD.
Carlisle St., Sheffield 4.

HERBERT MORRIS LTD.
P.O. Box 7, Loughborough, Leics.
THOMAS MORSON & SON, LTD.
Summerfield Chemical Works, Wharf Road, Enfield, Middx.
MOTIVITY
63 Park Road, Hampton Hill, Middx.
MUNDET CORK & PLASTICS LTD.
Vicarage Works, Vicarage Road, Croydon, Surrey.
A. W. MUNNS & CO., LTD.
63 Lincoln's Inn Fields, London, W.C.2.
TRADE AGENT FOR MYSORE IN LONDON
199 Piccadilly, London, W.1.

N

'NAARDEN' (LONDON) LTD.
73 Upper Richmond Rd., Putney, London, S.W.15.
NATIONAL ADHESIVES LTD.
Galvin Road, Slough, Bucks.
NATURAL & SYNTHETIC PERFUMERY ESSENCE CO.
108 City Road, London E.C.1.
NEALIS HARRISON LTD.
Courtney Street, Hull, Yorkshire.
NEUMO LTD.
South Coast Road, Peacehaven, Sussex.
THE NEW CONSOLIDATED MINES OF CORNWALL LTD.
Fairmead House, St. Austell, Cornwall.
NIPA LABORATORIES LTD.
Treforest Industrial Estate, Pontypridd, Glam.
NORDA-SCHIMMEL INTERNATIONAL LTD.
Stirling Road, Slough, Bucks.
NOVADEL LTD.
St. Ann's Crescent, London, S.W.18.

O

ORMCO LTD.
Ibex House, Minories, London, E.C.3.
ORMERODS LTD.
Hanging Road, Rochdale, Lancs.
D. J. OSBORNE CO., LTD.
72–76 Bensham Grove, Thornton Heath, Surrey.
OSBORNE, GARRETT, NAGELE LTD.
51/55 Frith St., London, W.1.

P

W. & C. PANTIN LTD.
Centre Drive, Epping, Essex.
THE PATENT BORAX CO., LTD.
Californian Works, Tipton, Staffs.
PATON CALVERT & CO., LTD.
Binns Road, Old Swan, Liverpool 13.
P. P. PAYNE & SONS, LTD.
Haydn Road, Nottingham.
L. R. B. PEARCE LTD.
125 High Holborn, London, W.C.1.
PEARSON & CO. (CHESTERFIELD), LTD.
The Potteries, Whittington Moor, Chesterfield.
PEERLESS & ERICSSON
1 Carlisle Road, The Hyde, London, N.W.9.
PEERLESS GOLD LEAF CO., LTD.
Fairfield Works, Bow, London, E.3.
PENNSALT LTD.
Tower Works, Doman Road, Camberley, Surrey.
P. T. PETLEY & CO. LTD.
9 St. Cross Street, London, E.C.1.
PFIZER, LTD.
Sandwich, Kent.
PHARMACAL SUPPLIES LTD.
Green Lane, Hounslow, Middx.
PHARMACEUTICAL LANOLINE CO.
17 Carnwath Road, London, S.W.6.
PIGALLE (INTERNATIONAL) LTD.
983 Finchley Road, London, N.W.11.
GEO. H. POOLE & SON (BOOTLE), LTD.
Canal Street Chemical Works, Bootle 20, Lancs.
POTH, HILLE & CO. LTD.
37 High St., Stratford, London, E.15.
A. V. POUND & CO., LTD.
Kemp House, 154/158 City Road, London, E.C.1.
PRATCHITT BROS. LTD. (Incorporated in LAM GROUP)
Denton Ironworks, Carlisle, Cumberland.
PREMIER COLLOID MILLS LTD.
Hersham Trading Estate, Walton-on-Thames, Surrey.
PREMIER OIL & CAKE MILLS LTD.
Stoneferry, Hull, Yorks.
PRICE'S (BROMBOROUGH) LTD.
Bebington, Wirral, Cheshire.
PRINTAR INDUSTRIES LTD.
Prince Regent's Wharf, Silvertown, London, E.16.
L. E. PRITCHITT & CO. LTD.
262 Uxbridge Road, Hatch End, Middx.
PROCTER & GAMBLE LTD.
G.P.O. Box 1 SH Newcastle-upon-Tyne 1.

PROCTER JOHNSON & CO. LTD.
Excelsior Works, Bank St., Clayton, Manchester, 11.
PRODORITE LTD.
Eagle Works, Wednesbury, Staffs.
PRONK, DAVIS & RUSBY LTD.
44 Penton St., London, N.1.
PROPRIETARY PERFUMES LTD.
International Perfumery Centre, Ashford, Kent.
PURFINOL LTD.
Petrofina House, York Road, London, S.E.1.

Q

QUICKFIT & QUARTZ LTD.
Tilling Drive, Stone, Staffs.
Q.V.F. LTD.
Duke Street, Fenton, Stoke-on-Trent, Staffs.

R

C. E. RAMSDEN & CO., LTD.
Foley Chemical Works, Fenton, Stoke-on-Trent, Staffs.
R. RAMSDEN & SON, LTD.
Faverdale, Darlington, Co. Durham.
WM. RANSOM & SON, LTD.
Hitchin, Herts.
RECKITT'S (COLOURS) LTD.
Morley St., Hull.
REEVES & SONS, LTD.
Lincoln Road, Enfield, Middx.
RELIANCE TRADING CO.
23–25 Charles Lane, St. John's Wood, London, N.W.8.
RENSHAM & ROMLEY LTD.
10 Canfield Place, London, N.W.6.
A. REVAI & CO. (CHEMICALS), LTD.
7–8 Idol Lane, London, E.C.3.
DAVID ROBERTS & SON
854 High Road, Tottenham, London, N.17.
ROBINSON BROS. LTD.
Ryders Green, West Bromwich, Staffs.
ROBINSON & SONS, LTD.
Wheat Bridge Mills, Chesterfield, Derbyshire.
E. S. & A. ROBINSON LTD.
Bristol.
ROCHE PRODUCTS LTD.
15 Manchester Square, London, W.1.
RONSHEIM & MOORE LTD.
140 Buckingham Palace Road, London, S.W.1.
ROSE, DOWNS & THOMPSON LTD.
Cannon Street, Hull, Yorks.
ROSE FORGROVE LTD.
432 Dewsbury Road, Leeds 11.

ROURE BERTRAND FILS ET JUSTIN DUPONT
63 Lincolns Inn Fields, London, W.C.2.
ROYLES LTD.
Irlam, Manchester.
H. RUBECK LTD.
9 St. Cross Street, London, E.C.1.

S

P. SAMUELSON & CO., LTD.
44–48 Paul Street, London, E.C.2.
SANDEMAN BROS. LTD.
50 Bilsland Drive, Maryhill, Glasgow.
H. G. SANDERS & SON, LTD.
Gordon Road, Southall, Middx.
ARTHUR SANDERSON & SONS, LTD.
52–53 Berners St., London, W.1.
SANDOZ PRODUCTS LTD.
P.O. Box Horsforth No. 4, Calverley Lane, Horsforth, Leeds.
R. SARANT & CO., LTD.
Napier House, 28–30 Second Cross Road, Twickenham, Middx.
R. P. SCHERER LTD.
216–222 Bath Road, Slough, Bucks.
A. & V. SCHULZE
60 High Street, Barnet, Herts.
GEORGE SCOTT & SON (LONDON), LTD.
Artillery House, Artillery Row, London, S.W.1.
SCOTT BADER & CO., LTD.
Wollaston, Wellingborough, Northants.
SCOTTISH FLAVOUR & COLOUR CO., LTD.
27–29 Ratcliffe Terrace, Edinburgh, Scotland.
SCOTTISH TAR DISTILLERS LTD.
Lime Wharf Chemical Works, Falkirk, Scotland.
MASSON SEELEY & CO., LTD.
137–139 Euston Road, London, N.W.1.
SELMAN & SON, LTD.
High Street, Earls Barton, Northamptonshire.
ANTHONY J. SHARP
1–3 Belmont Road, Whitstable, Kent.
THE SHARPLES COMPANY–A DIVISION OF PENNSALT LTD.
Tower Works, Doman Road, Camberly, Surrey.
SHEARMAN & CO., LTD.
Abbotskerswell, Newton Abbott, Devon.
SHELL CHEMICALS (U.K.) LTD.
Industrial Chemicals Division, Shell Centre, Downstream Building, London, S.E.1.
SHERMAN CHEMICALS LTD.
Downham Mills, Chestnut Road, Tottenham, London, N.17.

HENRY SIMON LTD.
Cheadle Heath, Stockport, Cheshire.
RICHARD SIMON & SONS, LTD.
Phoenix Works, Vernon Road, Basford, Nottingham.
W. S. SIMPSON & CO. (THE BRITISH ANILINE DYE & CHEMICAL WORKS) LTD.
1–23 Linden Way, London, N.14.
SIPON PRODUCTS LTD.
193–197 Regent Street, London, W.1.
A. J. SIRIS PRODUCTS LTD.
Lanchester, Co. Durham.
H. C. SLINGSBY LTD.
89–97 Kingsway, London, W.C.2.
SMITH & FORREST (OILS) LTD.
Holt Town Oil Works, Manchester 10.
SMITH & McLAURIN LTD.
Cartside Mills, Milliken Park, Renfrewshire.
WILFRID SMITH (FINE CHEMICALS) LTD.
Gemini House, High Street, Edgware, Middlesex.
SOFLOR LTD.
9 Wadsworth Road, Perivale, Greenford, Middx.
SOLPORT BROS. LTD.
Portia House, Goring Street, Goring-by-Sea, Sussex.
SOUTHALL & SMITH LTD. NOW DRIVER SOUTHALL LTD.
Villa St. Works, Hockley, Birmingham.
PETER SPENCE & SONS, LTD.
Moorfield Road, Widnes, Lancs.
SPENCER & HALSTEAD LTD.
Ossett, Yorks.
SPICERS LTD.
83 Piccadilly, London, W.1.
STAFFORD ALLEN & SONS, LTD.
20–42 Wharf Road, London, N.1.
STAINLESS STEEL PUMPS LTD.
Finmere Road, Eastbourne, Sussex.
STANDARD SYNTHETICS LTD.
76 Glentham Road, Barnes, London, S.W.13.
STAVELEY CHEMICALS LTD.
Nr. Chesterfield.
J. M. STEEL & CO., LTD.
Kingsway House, Parade Road, Richmond.
STEELE & COWLISHAW LTD.
Cooper St., Hanley, Stoke-on-Trent, Staffs.
STELCON LTD.
Clifford's Inn, London, E.C.4.
HENRY C. STEPHENS LTD. (Formerly THE STEPHENS GROUP.)
100 Drayton Park, Highbury, London, N.5.
HUGH STEVENSON & SONS, LTD.
Errwood Park, Crossley Road, Manchester 19.

STEVENSON & HOWELL LTD.
Standard Works, Southwark St., London, S.E.1.

COLIN STEWART LTD.
Central Offices, Wharton Hall, Winsford, Cheshire.

STOCKPACK LTD.
Corporation Street, Portwood, Stockport.

F. J. STOKES CO. & F. J. STOKES INTERNATIONAL (DIVISIONS OF PENNSALT LTD.)
Tower Works, Doman Road, Camberley.

STOKES & SMITH CO.
Belmont Works, St. Albans, Herts.

STOTHERT & PITT LTD.
Lower Bristol Road, Bath, Somerset.

STREETLEY MANUFACTURING CO., LTD.
Sutton Coldfield, Warwickshire.

H. E. STRINGER LTD.
Tring, Herts.

JOHN & E. STURGE LTD.
1 Wheeleys Road, Birmingham 15.

SURFASTAL LTD.
123 Bradford St., Birmingham 12.

SUTLEY & SILVERLOCK
31 Wilbury Way, Hitchin, Herts.

SYNTHITE LTD.
Ryders Green, West Bromwich, Staffs.

J. C. THOMPSON & CO. (DURON), LTD.
Duron Works, Drummond Road, Bradford, Yorks.

J. THOMPSON (DUDLEY) LTD.
Windmill Works, Dudley, Worcs.

JOHN THOMPSON-KENNICOTT LTD.
Ettingshall, Wolverhampton, Staffs.

3M CO., LTD.
3M House, Wigmore Street, London, W.1.

TITANIUM INTERMEDIATES LTD.
10 Stratton Street, London, W.1.

TOMLINSONS (ROCHDALE) LTD.
Oldham Road, Rochdale, Lancs.

TORRANCE & SONS, LTD.
Bitton, Nr. Bristol.

TOWNSON & MERCER LTD.
101 Beddington Lane, Croydon, Surrey.

H. TRAMER LTD.
Fleming Road, Speke, Liverpool, 24.

R. C. TREATT & CO., LTD.
19 Watling St., London, E.C.4.

TWEEDY OF BURNLEY LTD.
Gannow Lane, Burnley, Lancs.

JOHN TYE & SON, LTD.
The Sachet Centre, Gallows Corner, Romford, Essex.

TYRUPLEX LTD.
414–414A Harrow Road, London, W.9.

T

TAR RESIDUALS LTD.
Plantation House, Mincing Lane, London, E.C.3.

TAYLOR BROTHERS & COX LTD.
Adelaide House, King William St., London, E.C.4.

E. F. TAYLOR & CO., LTD.
Ampthill Road, Bedford.

TAYLOWE LTD.
Malvern Road, Furze Platt, Maidenhead, Berks.

TEAM VALLEY BRUSH CO.
Team Valley Trading Estate, Gateshead 11, Co. Durham.

THERMAL SYNDICATE LTD.
P.O. Box No. 6, Wallsend, Northumberland.

THEW, ARNOTT & CO., LTD.
Flodden Works, 270 London Road, Wallington, Surrey.

THEWS LTD.
Lustra Works, Soho Square, Liverpool 3.

THOMPSON BROS. (BILSTON) LTD.
Bradley Engineering Works, Bilston, Staffs.

U

UDEC LTD.
Cumberland Avenue, Park Royal, London, N.W.10.

UNGERER LTD.
14–18 Talacre Road, London, N.W.5.

UNION CARBIDE LTD. (CHEMICALS DIVISION)
P.O. Box 2 L.R., 8 Grafton St., London, W.1.

UNION GLUE & GELATINE CO. LTD.
Cransley Works, Garrett St., Golden Lane, London, E.C.1.

UNITED COKE & CHEMICALS LTD.
P.O. Box 136, Sales Dept., Handsworth, Sheffield, 13.

'UNIVER' (U.K. agents for MAURICE CHEVALIER)
24 High Holborn, London, W.C.1.

UNIVERSAL EMULSIFIERS LTD.
Invicta Works, 157 Mill St., East Malling, Kent.

UNIVERSAL OIL CO., LTD. THE
Oak Road, Clough Road, Hull, Yorks.

V

VELHO BLACKSTOCK & CO., LTD.
35a Aldersgate St., London, E.C.1.
VISCO LTD.
161 Stafford Road, Croydon, CR9 4DT.

W

JOHN WADDINGTON & SONS, LTD.
Wells Road, Guiseley, Leeds.
WADDINGTON & DUVAL (HOLDINGS) LTD.
Brewhouse Street, Putney, London, S.W.15.
THOS. WAIDE & SONS, LTD.
Kirkstall Hill, Leeds 5, Yorks.
STANLEY G. WALKER & CO., LTD.
Colour House, Manorgate Road, Kingston, Surrey.
THE WALKER CHEMICAL CO., LTD.
Liverpool Road, Warrington, Lancs.
WALKER CROSWELLER & CO., LTD.
Whaddon Works, Cheltenham, Glos.
WALLACH BROS. LTD.
12–16 Westland Place, London, N.1.
WARD, BLENKINSOP & CO., LTD.
Fulton House, Empire Way, Wembley, Middlesex.
THOS. W. WARD LTD.
Albion Works, Savile St., Sheffield 4.
JAMES WEBSTER & BRO. LTD.
Webster House, 163 Derby Road, Bootle, Liverpool 20.
WESTBROOK LANOLIN CO.
Daisy Bank, Duckworth Lane, Bradford, Yorks.
WESTWOOD MACNEILL & CO., LTD.
70 Wellington Street, Glasgow, C.2.
GEO. M. WHILEY LTD.
Victoria Road, Ruislip, Middx.
ALFRED PAUL WHITE & SON
7 Campion Road, London, S.W.15.

WHITE SEA & BALTIC CO., P & I DANISCHEWSKY LTD.
8/9 Hayne Street, London, E.C.1.
WHITE TOMKINS & COURAGE LTD.
North Albert Works, Reigate, Surrey.
WILKINS, CAMPBELL & CO., LTD.
Britannia Works, West Drayton, Middx.
S. W. WILKINSON & CO., LTD.
Western Road, Leicester.
WILLIAMS (HOUNSLOW) LTD. (Formerly WILLIAMS ANSBACHER LTD.)
Greville House, Hibernia Road, Hounslow, Middx.
WILSON & MANSFIELD LTD.
48 Gresham St., London, E.C.2.
VICTOR WOLF LTD.
Victoria Works, Croft St., Clayton, Manchester 11.
HARRY B. WOOD LTD.
48 Princess St., Manchester 1.
WORTHINGTON-SIMPSON LTD.
Lowfield Works, Newark, Notts.
WRIGHT BINDLEY & GELL LTD.
Percy Road, Greet, Birmingham 11.
WYNMOUTH LEHR & FATOILS LTD.
158 City Road, London, E.C.1.

Y

YORK SHIPLEY LTD.
North Circular Road, London, N.W.2.

Z

ZACH CARTWRIGHT LTD.
61/62 Crutched Friars, London, E.C.3.
A. & M. ZIMMERMANN
3 Lloyds Avenue, London, E.C.3.
CHAS. ZIMMERMANN & CO., LTD.
Pega Works, Walmgate Road, Perivale, Middx.

Further Reading

PERFUMES, COSMETICS AND SOAPS, W. A. Poucher. Chapman and Hall, London.

THE CHEMISTRY AND MANUFACTURE OF COSMETICS, M. G. de Navarre. Van Nostrand Reinhold Co. Ltd, New York and Wokingham, England.

MODERN COSMETICOLOGY, R. G. Harry. Leonard Hill Ltd, London.

These advanced books are recommended for readers who wish to study cosmetics in technical detail.